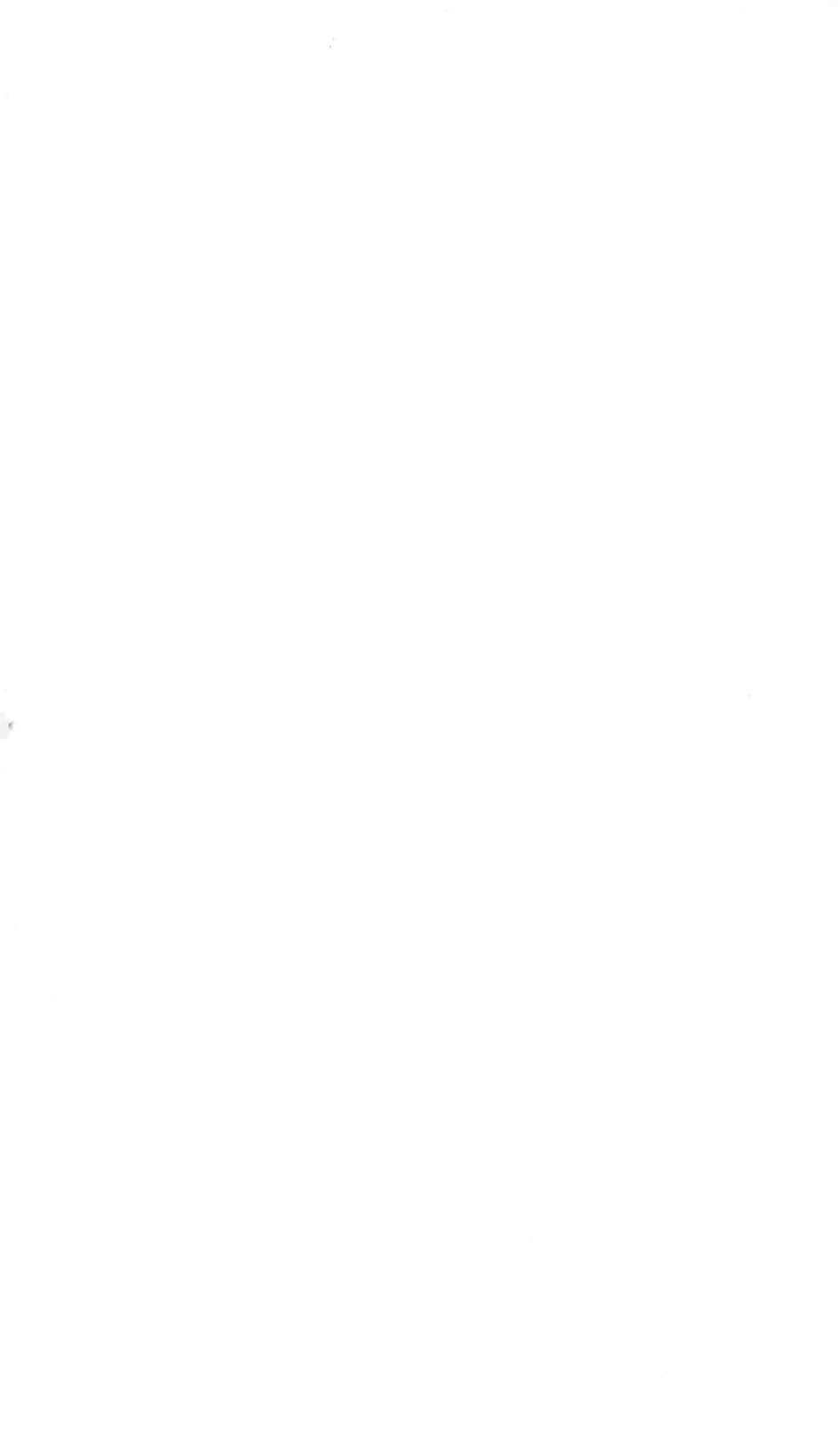

Under My Skin

Under My Skin

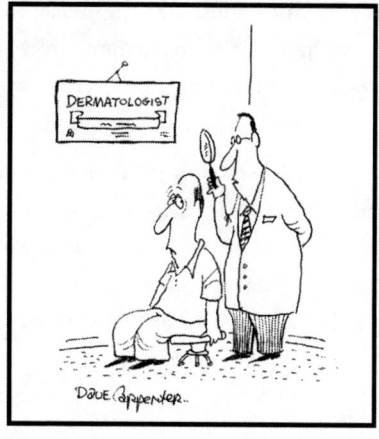

A Dermatologist Looks at His Profession and His Patients

Alan Rockoff, MD

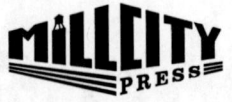

Mill City Press, Inc.

212 3rd Avenue North, Suite 290

Minneapolis, MN 55401

612.455.2294

www.millcitypublishing.com

ISBN-13: 978-1-937600-02-0

LCCN: 2011938399

Cover Design and Typeset by Wendy Baker

Dave Carpenter illustration courtesy of www.CartoonStock.com.

Printed in the United States of America

For Shuli

Contents

Foreword

For several years I have enjoyed reading Dr. Rockoff's monthly *Under My Skin* column in *Skin & Allergy News,* an independent magazine read by dermatologists across the United States. Dr. Rockoff's warm, wise, and witty reflections will resonate with every practicing physician, whether specializing in skin disease or otherwise engaged.

Dr. Rockoff's essays are always thoughtful, though his take can range in tone from deadpan to genial to laugh-out-loud hilarious. Underlying all his observations is the recognition that beneath the oddities, frustrations, and occasional small triumphs of daily practice lie the worries of ordinary people who have come for help and reassurance and, above all, to feel better. While addressing these needs, doctors have to deal with frustrating insurers, meddlesome bureaucrats, pharmaceutical salespeople, and professional pressures that may distract from immediate patient needs when they don't clash with them outright.

Dr. Rockoff addresses the tensions among these competing considerations. His rueful or humorous comments—always riveting—are also often bracing and cathartic. I hope this collection reaches a wide audience, not just of dermatologists, but of other medical professionals who devote their lives to caring for people. They are sure to find what Dr. Rockoff has to say useful, thought-provoking, and also delightfully entertaining.

In short, what has gotten under his skin has most certainly gotten under mine!

—Jerome Z. Litt, MD
Assistant Clinical Professor of Dermatology
Case Western Reserve University School of Medicine
Cleveland, Ohio

Preface

I became a dermatologist by accident.

The thought of joining the skin field never entered my mind in medical school, where I was taught nothing about it. Skin disease, in any case, seemed tangential to real medicine.

At my school real medicine meant Internal Medicine, our most prestigious department. I chose that discipline as my first required clinical rotation after the preclinical years of textbook study. Each day I trudged off to our large New York City Municipal Hospital, terrified I would fail to draw blood from my assigned patients and be mocked by all the bright house officers for whom aggressive ridicule seemed the core of departmental esprit.

On hospital rounds each morning these same assertive interns and residents vied with each other to show off their erudition. Fellow students, aiming to emulate and someday join them, rattled off the most recent data from the best journals. Intimidated, I kept my mouth shut.

Even more terrifying were the patients on our large, open wards. After spending the first two years of school thinking I had every disease our professors taught us about, I could now see actual patients sick and dying.

Terror leaves lasting impressions. I recall the Italian man in a twelve-bed room, surrounded by his large and attentive family. They could not console him in his last days as he lay oblivious, crying out for his Mama. The rooms farthest down the hall were set aside for patients who either needed less care or for whom there was nothing to do. On rounds, we passed without comment the private room in which patients admitted for terminal cancer passed their short sojourn. I sometimes gazed through the room's slightly open door at the bent, shriveled figure about whom our rounding entourage had nothing useful to say. And then there was Mrs. Fishkin, perky and cheerful despite what we then called senility. "Are you hungry?" the resident would ask. "Vell," she said with a whimsical smile, "I could eat."

In the end I chose to enter pediatrics. Sick children were somehow less threatening, and pediatricians seemed more easygoing than the internists I'd met. After training I took a job at a small Hartford hospital affiliated with the university. My position carried a grand-sounding title: Assistant Chief of Pediatrics. I felt all grown up. A month later, my boss sat me down and asked, "What do you want to do?"

I was naïve enough to think I was already doing it, but he set me straight.

"This is an entry-level job," he explained, "to introduce yourself to the community. The question is whether you want private practice or academics."

"Academics," I said, without conviction.

"In that case," he said, "you need a gimmick. Our department's sub-specialty needs are GI and Derm. Which would you like?"

Having never given a moment's thought to either, I chose dermatology. He then referred me to his friend and former pediatric colleague Sidney Hurwitz, down the road in New Haven. I spent parts of many Wednesdays with that remarkable and energetic man, then returned to home base and pretended to be a skin specialist. That I knew a bit more about skin than the people around me was both true and not very meaningful. One day I tried to use an old Hyfrecator-brand electric needle that was lying around the clinic; as pediatric residents watched in amazement, I pressed the footswitch and shocked myself across the room and against the wall. I regained my feet, and composure, with difficulty.

Two years later our hospital lost its academic affiliation. My halfhearted attempts to join a pediatric practice in town proved futile. Pediatricians need babies, but the residents of the Connecticut Valley were at that time busy implementing Zero Population Growth.

My wife, three small kids, and I moved to Boston, where I trained in dermatology and opened an office nearby. Hardly anyone opens solo practices anymore, and those who join groups build up their patient base much faster than I did. It took me five years to drop the last of eleven part-time jobs at various neighborhood health centers.

I often ask my patients how they came to do what they're doing.

Invariably they begin, "It was an accident..." Rather than heading straight from ambition to implementation, careers often trace a jagged path, the line of choice bent by sociology and nudged by contingency. "I knew this guy, there was this opening...and, somehow, here I am."

A few years ago the US government brought to town a national group of ambitious high-school students bent on medical careers. The kids got to meet physicians in academia, industry, and private practice. My story of how I got where I was didn't please them. They wanted a more coherent and inspirational narrative: seeing Dad's psoriasis spurred me to a life as a healer of the skin, that sort of thing. One seventeen-year-old from LA, nattily turned out in a cream-colored suit, handed me his business card.

Like everything else, the profession of medicine has changed a lot in the last thirty-two years. For one thing, we are far more consumer-oriented. You know that advertising no longer carries any stigma when academic teaching hospitals promote themselves like auto companies or department stores. "Our Primary Doctors Care About You!" says the ad in the Sunday health care section, along with a photo of smiling doctors who obviously care. "We Are #1 in Nephrology!" proclaims the banner in the hospital lobby. "Our Orthopedic Center Will Get You Back on the Golf Course in No Time!" says the TV ad. There is no point in lamenting the passing of old, paternalistic ways, but the new consumer culture does tend to change patients to clients and finally to customers, with complex consequences. While pondering these, you can always explore new ways to redesign your website and promote Search Engine Optimization.

The Internet, of course, changes everything. Anyone now has instant access to medical information from sources digested and reliable and others less so, as well as to consumer "reviews" that lump professionals with restaurants, tradesmen, and electric beard-trimmers.

Dermatology too has changed a great deal in the past three decades. Managed care, just getting started when I did, is now pervasive. An alphabet soup of government agencies and insurers exercises minute oversight of aspects of medical practice that used to be left to professional discretion: billing, occupational safety, patient privacy, and much more.

There are new sunscreens that actually don't wash off. Though they never used to, patients now come in for annual skin checks, and of course for cosmetic advice and procedures. Whether or not they have rashes or skin spots, people who visit a dermatology practice now expect to get skin care advice and find an array of techniques to help them look better and younger: laser removal of age spots or unwanted hair, chemical peels, cosmetic surgical procedures that range from an injection of Botox and fillers for wrinkles and furrows to eye lifts and neck tightening.

Those who choose to pay out of pocket for cosmetic work have different mindsets and expectations from those who are after more conventional medical advice. Often enough the same people come for one, then ask for the other, expressing themselves one way in the medical room and differently across the hall on the cosmetic side. In this as in so much else, people are endlessly paradoxical and fascinating. I will never fathom them—us—but have no plans to stop trying.

There are no physicians among my close relatives; the clergy is our family business. My late father was a rabbi, as are both my sons. I have always thought of my own role in pastoral terms, applying theory—medical, not theological—to help people, many of whom have neither knowledge of nor interest in official theories of any kind. What they want is to feel better and believe that what happens to them makes some kind of sense.

Doing this kind of work requires empathy, patience, and a certain emotional distance. Many patients are a delight to work with and a pleasure to help; a few are deeply annoying and endlessly needy. That's what you get when you deal with people. Those who expect otherwise might be better off doing something else.

You never really know what a job or profession is like until you actually do it. Though I wasn't clever enough to realize it in advance, dermatology is a wonderful way to spend professional life. It offers a varied clinical diet, many chances to provide reassurance, treatments that often help, gratified patients, comfortable hours, good pay. Practicing it gives one a chance to meet all kinds of people with interesting backgrounds and stories too curious to invent. Perhaps best of all, it presents the not-infrequent opportunity to hear someone say, "I feel so much better!" even if there really hasn't been much to do besides listen and smile reassuringly.

Each day brings a swirl of patients, practitioners, staff, and clinical and administrative challenges. Sometimes I take a step back, think of the part-time jobs and the empty, two-room office of thirty years ago, and wonder how on earth I got here. Surely, personal choices played a role—they must have, mustn't they?—but it's hard to remember what those choices were and what effect they had.

Somehow, becoming a dermatologist still feels like an accident. A pleasant one.

• • • • •

I want to thank my editors at *Skin & Allergy News*, where many of these essays have appeared as columns. Special thanks to my current editor, Amy Pfeiffer, as well as to Richard Camer, the editor who first invited me to write a column called "Under My Skin" thirteen years ago.

Thanks to my dermatologic colleagues, for their e-mails of response and encouragement. Glad to know similar things happen in your offices.

Thanks to my patients, for sharing their lives and experiences along with their medical problems. From all who taught me I have learned.

I offer thanks to my parents, who claim not to remember encouraging me to be a doctor. My late father, Rabbi Irving Rockoff, taught me that people are what matter. My mother Betty Rockoff, about to turn ninety, reads everything I write. The magnificent needlepoint she made when I graduated medical school adorns one of my examining rooms, eliciting admiration from many patients, one of whom said, "Whoever did that must love you very much." (But Ma, why the golf clubs?)

My deep thanks to my children Yael, Aaron, and Daniel, for reading these columns as they appeared and for their comments, support, and love.

Most of all, thanks to my wonderful wife Shuli, for everything that matters.

PRACTICE

Starting Out

"Where should we go into practice?" With the end of training in sight, we residents pondered that question to the point of obsession. Salaried positions weren't popular in Boston in the late '70s. Those who aspired to professional life outside the academy either joined a group practice or went solo, still an option in those days.

I had heard about many groups that dissolved in acrimony. Most practitioners I knew worked alone. So would I.

But where? Everybody said that Boston had too many doctors, but maybe there was a niche somewhere around that wasn't filled yet. Whom could I ask for unbiased guidance? Sheltered professors wouldn't know. Fellow residents were as ignorant as I. Established practitioners were famous for less than full candor when counseling potential competitors.

Journal want-ads weren't much help either. They listed attractive opportunities in western Tennessee or central Minnesota, with ample scope for hunting, fishing, and a family-oriented outdoor lifestyle. Not what an urban-bred couple and three small children were after.

Dad lobbied for us to return to suburban New York. His friends told him, "Skin doctors cart their deposits to the bank in wheelbarrows." My wife and I hated to disappoint him, but we wanted no part of either Long Island or wheelbarrows. Instead we contemplated a move south.

Choosing at random from a specialist's directory, I called a doctor in Atlanta. He sounded depressed. "Five years ago there were thirty-seven dermatologists in our medical society," he said. "Now there are eighty, but only the same number of patients to go around."

The mood of a Washington, DC practitioner was just as downbeat. "Used to be you had to wait two weeks to get an appointment," he sighed. "Now I can see you this afternoon."

Prospects near home began to look brighter, if only by comparison. In the end I succumbed to inertia and chose to start a practice from scratch in the close-in suburb of Brookline. That was where we lived and had friends, where we knew the schools and stores to buy groceries. Colleagues were skeptical: didn't I know that if Boston was full of doctors, Brookline was choking on them? Hadn't I heard that Fred had opened in Brookline, then had to close and move to Cape Cod?

Sure, I'd heard about Fred, but I convinced myself that diligence, affability, and part-time clinic jobs would see me through. Besides, Fred was primarily a pathologist with a personality to match.

Having made a decision, I cast about for evidence to support it. I turned not to other dermatologists but to potential referring physicians, who I assumed would have no reason to feel threatened by my practice.

My first contacts were encouraging. I was exhilarated to find primary doctors who insisted that, despite the many dermatologists listed in the phone book, they "didn't know a single one." They could "hardly wait" for me to hang out my shingle. One suggested I contact a man I'll call Myron Drapkin, head of an allergy group just a few blocks from our apartment. "That's a huge practice," said my informant. "Myron can set you straight on the need for dermatologists around here."

Delighted at how clever my choice of staying put was starting to look, I called the allergist at once. He sounded most cordial and asked me to meet him after work the very next day.

With rare promptness I showed up at Drapkin's office, tense and a bit giddy. He stood waiting for me: 50-ish, graying at the temples, sporting a gray suit as understated as his office façade. Fixing me with an appraising gaze, he clasped my shoulder and said, "You look like a nice Jewish boy. Let's go have a drink."

Everyone at Walter's knew him. When we sat down, he told me I was doing the right thing. "You've got to get out and make contacts," he said. "You can't just sit on your duff and wait for patients to show up or for doctors to send them to you."

We sipped our beers. Drapkin went on in a meditative vein. He told me about his son, who had overcome dyslexia to graduate college; about his old house, which had expensive electric heat, and his new one, more economically outfitted with gas. Then his tone changed.

"We have a big allergy practice," he said. "People come long distances to see us, from all over Greater Boston. If one of them has a skin problem, could you accommodate him right away so he won't have to go home and return?"

Of course I could!

"That's good," he said. "We refer a lot of patients. You know Lewenthal, the internist down the street? We sent him dozens of patients when he opened up, and really put him on his feet. And there's an orthopedist at St. Joe's. Last year alone our office sent him seventy-four patients."

"Seventy-four?" I asked. "Do you keep score?"

"Oh yes," he said, "it's important, for us and our patients. When you open for business, be sure to come by and drop off some of your cards."

Ecstatic, I rushed home to tell my wife I'd struck the mother lode: dozens of patients from all over the area! I'd have to beat them off with a stick.

June came. With my two-room, subleased office equipped and ready, I called my anticipated benefactor. Drapkin's secretary said he was very busy. She set up a meeting for the following Monday, but Drapkin wasn't there when I showed up. He'd forgotten the appointment.

Several tries later I arranged to meet on a weekday at noon. The allergist looked distracted, flashing me a vague smile that suggested I looked somehow familiar. I handed him a packet of my brand-new embossed cards showing my name, address, and telephone number, along with the brave words, "By Appointment" (as if I'd turn away a walk-in).

Tossing aside the cards, Drapkin motioned for me to sit opposite at his cluttered desk. With an absent gaze he started to speak.

"Let me tell you a story," he said. "When I started practice, an older doctor promised to send me a lot of referrals. Weeks and months went by, but not a single one came. The man tried to avoid me in the hospital and at medical society meetings, but one day he couldn't.

"'Look,' he said, 'I'm embarrassed. I promised to send you patients, and I haven't.'

"No need to apologize,' I told him. 'You don't owe me anything.' That's just what I said, and I meant it too. No hard feelings."

Then Drapkin looked straight at me. "You just get out there, knock on doors, introduce yourself, hand out cards. Good luck. But just remember what I told that doctor and what I'm telling you. Nobody owes anybody anything."

On July 1 I sent out announcements, opened my doors, and waited. For a long time my only regular referral source was the Yellow Pages. As time passed patients trickled in, brought by word of mouth or sent by doctors who, for one reason or another, took an occasional break from the specialists they usually used. As for those who had said they could hardly wait for me to open my doors, I never heard from most of them again.

Drapkin did eventually call, about four years later. It seems he had a patient with a skin problem who had traveled from a far corner of the metropolitan area. Would I accommodate him by seeing the patient right away?

Of course I would. Considering his kind referral and the valuable lesson he'd taught me, it was the least I could do.

I Googled You

When I started practice, patients found me through the Yellow Pages. "I recognized your address," they said. "You were convenient." It seemed a little impersonal, but what could I expect? I was new.

Later, patients found me on HMO lists. Their physicians referred them because at the time I was the only dermatologist on the insurance rosters, my older colleagues having refused to join on principle. I dutifully sent referral letters to physicians I didn't know. "Dear Doctor X. Thank you for referring Jane. I am treating her acne with such-and-such." Perhaps someone read them.

As my reputation grew, I began getting referrals from doctors' receptionists. "They gave me a list," patients would say. 'Here are the three dermatologists we use. The lady at the front desk suggested you.'

I understood all this. Even before our field became synonymous in the public mind with Botox and cosmetic fluff, non-dermatologists thought of skin disease as something exotic and superficial ("It's one of those skin things. Go see a skin guy."), if not alien and frightening ("Lordy, it's one of those skin things! Go see a skin guy!").

Perhaps I'm wrong, but I can't imagine similar referrals to other specialties. ("Your ticker is tocking. Go see a heart guy.") In any case, even when patients have come from other physicians, I have rarely felt a sense of the real collegiality that I imagine takes place in hospital corridors and cafeterias. Once in a great while over the years, I've gotten an urgent call from a doctor in my own building eager to send down a patient with a dramatic rash, or even gone upstairs myself while the patient was still with the internist or surgeon. Such occasions have been uniquely satisfying, though rare enough that I can actually remember them.

Now that I've been around for a long time, many of the doctors who used to send me patients have retired, slowed down, or gone concierge. Also, more people are insured by PPO's that don't require physician referral. As a result, when I ask, "Who referred you to me?" I'm apt to hear, "I looked you up online on my insurer's website, and I recognized your address. You were convenient." Higher-tech, but familiar.

Sometimes people are referred by other people. "I got your name from a friend," they'll say.

"Neat. Which friend?"

"Uhhh…actually, I think it was my mother-in-law's friend."

Then of course there's Google. "I did an Internet search," a new patient says.

"No kidding," I reply. "What did you search for?"

"Dermatologists in Brookline."

Makes you feel warm and fuzzy all over, doesn't it?

One patient was more flattering. "I Googled 'Top Dermatologists, Brookline.'"

Wow, I thought. I've been Optimized.

I Googled that myself, and what came up first was an Internet Yellow Pages site with a list headed by "Featured Advertisers: Dermatology." The first of these was an animal hospital with a special offer: "Get coupon for Pet's first visit!" Below that was a listing for a (human) dermatologist in a town twenty miles north. Scrolling down past more advertisers and a long paragraph of skin-related keywords, there were actual dermatologists in Brookline. I came in second among these, with an incorrect address.

Just for fun, I Googled, "Bottom Dermatologist Brookline." The first listing for that was an answer on a medical website I wrote five years ago to a worried questioner who had pimples on his bottom. Bottom's up!

A while back I saw a patient who identified herself as a "health writer for the *Wall Street Journal*." After I examined her, she asked me for the name of an internist. "I need someone affiliated with a major teaching hospital," she said. "In case I get sick, I need access to the most advanced medical care. I'm a sophisticated medical consumer," she added. "After all, I'm a health writer for the *Wall Street Journal*."

I gave her the names of two doctors. "By the way," I asked, "how did you find me?"

"The mailman," she said. "I met him while I was walking by your building, and he told me he hears you're good."

Well, I am the only dermatologist in the building.

Instructions

My associate, Kate, gave Chris a prescription for a medicated wash and asked him to use it twice a day. Chris looked annoyed.

"Hold on," he said. "You didn't tell me how to use it."

This flummoxed Kate. "You...wash with it," she said.

"You said twice a day, but you didn't say when."

"Morning and night."

"After a shower?"

"That would be one good time."

"Do I put it on with my fingers, or do I have to use a cloth or a cotton swab?"

"Fingers are fine."

"And then do I wash it off, or leave it there?"

"It's a wash, Chris," Kate told him. "You wash it off."

Although Chris may have been a bit more anxious and unclear on the concept than most, his fusillade of questions differs from that of many patients only in degree. A lot of instructions obvious to doctors are a whole lot less so to people we give them to.

From sometimes challenging experience, I offer this non-exhaustive list of instructions intended to address questions before they're asked:

Oral medication:

1. <u>Take this pill twice a day, morning and night</u>. Not as obvious as it sounds, as becomes clear when people ask, "Wait, which two times?" I am sometimes tempted to say, "7:16 a.m. and 9:18 p.m. Sharp!" But I don't.

2. <u>Take it with food (or on an empty stomach)</u>. Even if it doesn't really matter, being specific and decisive helps the anxious.

3. <u>You can take it together with other medications</u>. This isn't self-evident either. Patients suspect that taking several pills at the same time will compromise the safety and effectiveness of each, or somehow overwhelm their system ("Won't it be too much for me?"). If they think they have to wait between their various medications, they may skip one and forget to take it later.

4. <u>Space the doses out during waking hours</u>. Many people ignore instructions. Others follow them too closely: say "four times a day," and they set their alarms for 2 a.m.

Topical (external, not tropical) medication:

5. <u>Apply it twice a day, morning and night.</u> See #1.

6. <u>Put it on when the skin is damp (or dry, or whatever)</u>. Again, many patients, especially the elderly, need specificity. Leaving things to their discretion just makes them nervous.

7. <u>You can put lotion or makeup on right on top of the medication</u>. Not at all obvious, since patients assume that another cream (or clothing) will "rub off" the medication and negate it. On the pitfalls of having to wait for whatever comes next in the daily skin care regimen, see # 3.

8. <u>Wash the medication off (for washes). Leave the medication on (for creams and lotions)</u>. For scalp dandruff, for example, it may be unclear to many patients that they should shampoo— *and wash it off*—and then apply a cortisone lotion, *and leave it on*. ("Wait, could you repeat that, Doc?")

9. <u>Apply the acne treatment all over the face, not just on the spots</u>.

10. <u>You can put the cream on with your fingers</u>. The fastidious prefer cotton, which is fine, but harder to use if you want to rub the cream in fully.

These examples apply to patients in general, but some, like the stars of the following mini-dramas, are more than usually clueless. Supply your own rim-shots after each:

* * * * *

"Thanks for showing me how to pop open the tube and apply the cream, Doctor, but my rash is on my leg and you put the cream on the back of your hand. Should I put it on my hand?"

"No, you put it on your rash."

* * * * *

Where do I get this medication?"

"In a pharmacy."

"Any pharmacy?"

"Yes."

* * * * *

And my personal favorite. (An actual case, honest!)

"What do I do when I run out of cream?"

"Go to the pharmacy for a refill."

"How do they refill it?"

"They give you more."

"I don't get it, Doctor—how do they get the cream back into the crumpled-up tube?"

AAARRRGGGHHH!!!!!!!!

The Cream Won't Rub Off

Doctors Are from Mars, Patients Are from Duluth

The back of my left hand is free of acne and eczema, because that is where I show patients how to apply topical antibiotic and steroid creams, adding:

"Rub it in thinly, like this. Twice a day, in the morning after you wash and at bedtime. And remember—once you rub the cream in, it attaches to your skin and won't come off if you wash later on or if clothing rubs against it."

This small lesson often brings a nod of understanding, as though I said something unusually wise. Unless you tell people the cream won't come off, they assume that it will rub off and that there's therefore no point in putting it on. It took me years to figure this out, as I pondered exchanges like these with Smith and Jones, two patients with hand eczema.

Sorry, Doc, I put that cortisone cream on in the morning like you told me, but I couldn't put it on at night. It would just come off on the sheets.

Were you afraid it would mess up your bedclothes, Mrs. Smith?

No, it's not greasy or anything. But it would just come off.

Roll that around your frontal lobes a little. What does it mean to say that the cream would "come off?" And why should whatever it means imply that it's better not to put it on in the first place? While you're thinking about those matters, consider Jones:

My feet are always dry and cracked, Doctor. I apply Vaseline and wear white cotton socks all night, but in the morning I'm still dry.

Two questions: Why do the gloves have to be white? And more to the point at hand (or at foot), why wear gloves at all?

For a long time, in my clunky, physicianly way, I thought in functional terms: the Vaseline would mess up the pillow, etc. It took me many years and a few drinks to loosen up my brain connections, break out of my conceptual box, and get some insight into Smith's noncompliance and Jones's white gloves:

To patients, creams are easy come, easy go. Your fingers rub them in, and clothes or water rub them right off. Applying cream and then putting on a pair of pants or slipping under the covers makes as much sense—to the patient—as taking a pill and spitting it out. Hold on! Does that mean that if a cream is going to come off, it's better not to put it on in the first place? You bet. Just ask Smith.

No matter how confident our manner or impressive our white coat, patients will find ways not to perform treatments that make no sense—to them. Medical advice can sound dangerous or silly for many reasons. When it comes to applying creams, for instance, we doctors are quantitative and analytical, but our patients are qualitative and holistic. We see cream absorption as a process one can measure: you can have all, a lot, or a little. To patients, however, it's all or nothing. Rubbing is rubbing. You rub once and it's on. Rub again and it's off.

Doctors needn't take my word for this. Next time they recommend a cream, they can add that once the cream is on, it won't rub off if water or clothes touch the skin. They can then watch the light go on:

Oh, I get it. Once I put the cream on, it won't come off! I didn't know that!

Medicines work so much better when people use them.

What about Jones's insistence on white gloves? White is the color of cleanliness and purity, while skin disease implies poor hygiene ("How can I have eczema? I wash every day!"), even defilement.

But that's a discussion for another time.

Mistakes

Jenna wanted to show me something on her upper lip. She and her young family were about to move to Berlin in five days. "This has been here for a year," she said. "I think it may have grown."

I stared at it in bright light with high magnification. "It looks like a large pore," I said. "It's small and perfectly round. I don't think it's a problem." I refilled her acne medication and wished her luck, suggesting that she e-mail me if she had any concerns after she got settled.

Two months later Jenna did just that, telling me that the spot on her lip had grown further. I sent her the names of dermatologists in Berlin. Shortly afterward she wrote me again. "What you said was a 'pore' is actually a basal cell skin cancer. I'm disappointed that it wasn't diagnosed earlier."

You would think that after all these years practicing dermatology I would recognize the most common form of skin cancer.

Everyone knows that humans make mistakes, but it's hard to admit that we are that particular human. This is true even if the mistake isn't likely to result in death or a lawsuit. Admitting fallibility is hard, especially for doctors, because being wrong is embarrassing. So often patients put us on a pedestal, whether we deserve to be up there or not, and it's tough to climb off.

In our professional role we are always calm and competent. People come to us when they're in trouble; they count on us to get things right. If we let them down, can they trust us the next time around? Can we trust ourselves?

The answer to whether they can trust us again is often, "No." Even after a warm clinical relationship spanning years, a missed diagnosis may be followed almost at once by a signed request to "Forward my records to…" It doesn't matter how many correct diagnoses came before, how many ultra-precautionary biopsies were negative—sometimes it's one strike and you're out. This may seem unfair, but it's really no more than the other side of the relationship: all that undeserved adulation. ("You're fantastic, Doctor! You gave me that cream five years ago, and my psoriasis never came back!")

Anyone in practice long enough gets his or her share of letters expressing anger or disappointment. Sending a self-justifying response is usually unhelpful, if not useless. But who among us is courageous—or foolish—enough to say, "Sorry, but you're right—I blew it"?

For dermatologists there are few errors we can make that have dire or irreversible consequences. Missing a melanoma is, of course, such a mistake. Yet despite hypervigilance, careful examination, and frequent biopsy, there will always be that funny lesion that doesn't look the way a melanoma is supposed to, about which the patient—or attorney—may later demand, "Can you explain why you didn't test that, Doctor?"

We might respond to errors or oversights with frustration, or a guilty conscience. Either way, it's hard to admit we came up short. Now and then a patient or relative will rub in our shortcomings with special relish.

Last year I diagnosed and treated a basal cell skin cancer on the forehead of an elderly Russian woman. She returned a few months later to show me another spot on her upper lip. "You said it was okay," she said, "but my daughter is worried." Although I could barely see the lesion, a biopsy confirmed that it, too, was a basal cell.

Her daughter, who turned out to be a family practitioner, called soon after. "Tell me," she said, her voice heavy with sarcasm, "when you look at the forehead, do you also look a few centimeters down to the lip, or is that too much trouble?"

Taken aback, I offered no response. "My mother has a daughter who is a physician," she went on. "What happens to your patients who don't have that luxury?"

I could have responded by hoping that if she herself ever makes an error, her patients might be more forbearing. But I said only that I understood her point.

As for Jenna, I answered her e-mail by saying that her lip lesion had not looked to me like a skin cancer and that I tried to avoid biopsies on the faces of young people when possible. I added that I was sure she would be well taken care of.

Hippocrates had it right: "Life is short, the art long, opportunity fleeting, experience misleading, judgment difficult." All we can do is keep trying.

You're Wonderful, Doctor!

The young woman I saw the other day was full of admiration. I had just burned off a wart on her shin.

"I can't believe it was so simple!" she exclaimed. "My friend who referred me said you were great, and she was right."

Why was I great? Because she had a wart and not a skin cancer? Because electric needles work?

"Always take credit," I tell students, "whether you deserve it or not, for most assuredly you will have to take blame the same way." That's my Ben Franklin mode.

It's true, though. We often get the credit when things go well, whether we deserve it or not. How many times has a returning acne patient enthused, "That antibiotic you prescribed is awesome! My zits were gone in three days."

Now we know perfectly well that antibiotics don't work for acne in three days, and what really happened is that we caught the wave of spontaneous improvement in a condition that by its nature goes up and down. But we aren't going to admit that, are we? Lose all that therapeutic transference? No way!

Actually, all of us, physicians and laymen alike, benefit from unmerited praise all the time. When someone says, "Your son is so tall and handsome!" we grow an inch ourselves and glow with pride. What are we proud of? Did we make him tall? Did we rearrange his features to conform to prevailing cultural norms? Yet we accept this praise as no less than what we deserve. (There were those expensive braces, anyway.)

The plain fact is that we get and take the credit when things go well, whether or not we had a meaningful hand in making them go that way.

There is, of course, a flip side, because here as elsewhere there is no free lunch. When things don't go well, we take the blame, deserved or not. We've all had the phone call. "It's Mrs. Goldfarb on Line 3," beeps the receptionist wearily. We approach the phone with resigned trepidation. Her third call this week, and it's only Tuesday. "How are you, Mrs. Goldfarb?" we say, trying to sound hopeful. Maybe finally…

Her grating tone lands like a pail of cold water. "Not good AT ALL, Doctor," she says, with emphasis. "What's the problem now?" we ask, as if we didn't know. "I'm still itching," she says, "and it's TERRIBLE. Yesterday I told you about my back. Now my left ankle itches. It kept me up all night…"

Diseases that by their nature don't get much better put a strain on the therapeutic relationship. Most patients want to cooperate by getting better. They feel that failure to do so means letting you down. We in turn recognize that not improving isn't their fault, but it's sometimes hard not to feel twinges of resentment toward people who, despite your best efforts, refuse to get well. We can suppress the urge to express this feeling, but no one can pretend it isn't there.

That's why dermatology is such a lovely field. The standard knock is that our patients never die and never get better, but that doesn't grasp the heart of the matter at all. The slice of clinical reality we deal with has many healthy people who worry about things we can reassure them about, who clear up or grow out of their acne, whose warts respond to treatment or go away by themselves, who get benign growths we can scrape off and cancers we can mostly cure. Of course not everything we deal with is so rosy, but most of our patients aren't miserable, or don't stay that way for long. Even most hives let up sooner or later.

And we benefit from this by taking credit: when we tell a gray-haired grandma that the irritation at the corner of her mouth isn't cancer and she beams us a look of beatitude; when a sweet young thing looks across at the bald, gray-bearded guy who's just zapped a wart off her shin and gushes, her eyes dewy with transference, "You're wonderful, Doctor!"

Is this a great specialty or what?

Short Notice

(9:30 a.m.)

"Doctor, thank you for seeing me on such short notice."

"When did you call for an appointment?"

"Two days ago."

"Sappho, in my office. Right now!"

"What's the matter, Doctor?"

"My last patient called only two days ago and got an appointment."

"But you had an opening…"

"I know it, and you know it, but the whole world doesn't have to know it. What if my colleagues find out? When do we get Grisnelda's Mystery Shopper report?"

"At lunch, today."

(12:20 p.m.)

"Okay, Grisnelda, whenever you're ready."

"As you instructed, Doctor, I made this quarter's calls to try getting appointments around town."

"Excellent, Grisnelda. Did you use the untraceable cellphone?"

"Yes, and then I threw it in the Charles River just like they do in the Hudson on *Law and Order*."

"Great, what did you find?"

"Borromeo Dermatology has a six-week wait, down from seven last quarter. Birkenstock Integrative Cutaneous Wellness has nine weeks, up from eight. Stanislavsky Skin is holding steady at four months."

"Stanislavsky only works Wednesday afternoons. What about the hospital clinics?"

"At Mount Saint Helen's they can see you in November."

"November of this year? By that time, you'll probably either be better or too sick to care."

"And then of course there's UADLPSSCADLE."

"Who on earth is that?"

"That's the new name for Metroderm, the big group with offices all over. It stands for "Urban Agglomeration for Dermatology, Laser, Plastic Surgery, Skin Care, Age Defiance, and Lifestyle Enhancement.""

"Good heavens, how do they answer the phone?"

"'Urban Agglomeration—where, to whom, and toward what end may we direct your call?' They have a three-month wait, and that's after dropping Medicaid and all the low-paying HMO's."

"We actually get some of their acne patients who take Isotretinoin. They need to be confirmed on the federal online registration program every month, but the office can't fit them in for follow-up in under two. Sappho, do you see how embarrassing this is? What kind of place must this practice be if you can be seen the day after tomorrow? Why would anybody want to get an appointment at a place where anybody can just call up and get an appointment?"

"But, Doctor…"

"Let me make this perfectly clear. If we let on that I have openings and the word gets out, then people will be unwilling to make appointments, and then I'll have openings. Do you follow?"

"Not exactly…"

"Well, thanks for your input, everybody. It's time to get back to work."

(3:15 p.m.)

"Good afternoon, Mrs. Rabinowitz. My goodness, I haven't seen you in four years."

"I had a problem last summer, Doctor, but you were on vacation, and they told me I wouldn't be able to see you for three months."

"Three months! Mrs. Rabinowitz, in more than thirty years I have never had patients wait anywhere near that long. In fact..."

"Well, that's what the receptionist told me, Doctor. So I called another dermatologist down the street, and he took care of me the same day. Such a nice young man, too."

Accentuate the Positive

It's best to never tell a patient she has a bad case. Even if just a case of pimples.

Consider Celia, who showed up at age twenty-five with severe acne. Nothing unusual about that.

"Have you ever seen a doctor about this?"

"Once, when I was sixteen," she said. "But it seems like yesterday. I was afraid to go to a dermatologist, but my mother finally dragged me. We were waiting, when he burst in to the room, took one look at me, and said, 'My God, your face is terrible!' I ran out crying," she concluded, "and I haven't ever gone back to a doctor about it."

If this were a rational world, Celia's behavior would make no sense. Granted, her dermatologist was brusque and insensitive. But shouldn't having a professional confirm that her case is severe make Celia even more eager to take care of it? Actually not.

In the world of consultants, people act to maximize their wealth, health, and ability to function. In the world of clinical practice, patients often do whatever they can to escape bad news, even to their own objective detriment. Doctors who don't watch our words and our body language can, without meaning to, help folks avoid getting better.

When examining the patient, we can, for instance, frown, look downcast, shake our heads, say or imply that things aren't going well, or say, "You have a bad case..."

Our training tells us to be objective, as indeed we must. If things aren't going well, we have to take steps to improve them. As for declaring that a case is bad, so what? A "bad case" of acne or eczema isn't going to kill her, is it? Besides, since she can see for herself the way things stand, why not confirm the obvious?

Because it makes her feel rotten, offended, and pessimistic. Objectively, our assessment changes nothing. Yet hearing someone in authority declare that things aren't going well makes everything feel worse.

Imagine you're at a party when an old acquaintance approaches, grinning. "Hello, old sport!" he booms. "Haven't seen you in years. You look splendid!"

Makes you feel like a million bucks, doesn't it? Puts a smile on your face and a spring in your step. But why should it? What's changed?

Now consider the opposite scenario. Your old pal looks worried. "Have you been ill?" he asks, with a slight tremolo. "You're pale. Sure you're all right?"

Well, you were till a minute ago. Right now you feel as though someone's kneed you in the gut. You duck out to find a mirror. Maybe you are a little sallow…

Again, why? Your blood pressure's the same, your blood count hasn't changed a whit. But you feel lousy anyway.

Telling patients things are "bad" has precisely this effect, whatever the objective situation. It's quite common, for instance, for a patient to ask about her rosacea, "Is it a *bad case*, Doctor?" A response like, "Why, no! It's quite a mild case, and we can take care of it!" produces a relieved facial expression that tells the tale.

Does any of this matter? Most certainly. Pessimistic patients skip appointments, stop treatment, and interpret every downturn as further proof of the futility of proceeding. The judgment, "You have a bad case," becomes a prophecy that fulfills itself.

The nineteenth-century French neurologist Paul Dubois, in his long-forgotten treatise, The Psychic Treatment of Nervous Diseases, put it this way:

When one has succeeded in inspiring the patient [with confidence of improvement], it is necessary to encourage this state of mind during the whole treatment. Every time that there is any fact detected which confirms the favorable prognosis, it should be commented on…All improvement, however slight it may be…should be noted, and the patient must draw new reasons for raising his courage from these proofs.

Cool objectivity belongs in chart notes and case reports. In the exam room, however, whether treating a new patient or managing the ups and downs of an old one, there's always something positive to say. It's best to find it, and say it.

Why Are You Prescribing That, Doc?

"I've had this groin rash for weeks," says Harry. "Dr. Skinflint's tried different creams." Harry dumps tubes from a plastic bag onto his lap. The first is for treating fungus, the second for eczema, the third for bacterial infections.

Good question: What was the doctor thinking?

Better question: What was the patient thinking?

Did Harry ask, "Gee, Doc, you gave me a fungus cream, then you switched to a steroid, and now it's an antibacterial. Do you have any idea what I have?" Harry did not ask this.

I am impressed, even amazed, at how often patients fail to ask doctors what we're doing and why. A college student from another state has taken an antibiotic to treat acne for two years, with no discernible effect. Has he asked his doctor, "Why are we staying with the same thing if it's not working?" He has not. Neither has his mother.

Of course, some people do ask; I don't mind explaining what I'm doing, and often do so at length until, not infrequently, I see the patient's eyes glaze over with the unspoken plea, "Could you please just give me the prescription so I can get out of here?"

This lack of inquisitiveness crosses socioeconomic lines. College profs and working stiffs seem equally unlikely to challenge therapeutic decisions by asking doctors to explain and justify them. I use the word "challenge" advisedly.

If we were presenting a case on hospital rounds, we would expect our senior physician to have us explain our treatment plan and to ask, "Why are you doing this, and how will it work?" When patients ask this way, however, the questioning often comes across more as a challenge to authority than a request for information, as in, "So how do I know you know what you're doing?" Few patients are aggressive enough to do that. Thank heavens.

We are trained to make the right diagnosis and prescribe the best treatment, based on the best available evidence. I am all for this, and do it whenever possible. But in daily clinical life, the diagnosis is often unclear, treatment options fuzzy, evidence for effectiveness limited.

It's a relief then when patients cut us slack and don't demand detailed explanations for many of our decisions. This comes in handy when we either don't have them or, for one reason or other, can't put them across.

I am not referring to high-stakes diagnostic and therapeutic challenges like exotic diseases, medical mysteries, or excruciating end-of-life issues. Such situations generate learned musings on the dynamics and ethics of doctor-patient communication. The examples I have in mind are more homely, even trivial: the kinds of things, in other words, we deal with every day.

Consider Archie, a three-year-old with infantile eczema. His mother insists that Archie "has been treated with everything," and that "nothing works." In this case Archie has indeed been treated appropriately with a series of steroids and non-steroids. Since the diagnosis is clear, it seems reasonable to assume that what Mom means by "nothing is working" is that nothing has worked completely, or fast enough, or prevented the rash from coming back elsewhere.

My own approach in such cases is to tell Mom, "I have a new and different cream that I'm convinced is just right for Archie." I ask that she apply it everywhere necessary twice a day, without fail, for ten days and return. It often turns out to work. Not because it is "better" by some objective standard but because she actually used it long enough to see a result. Now she'll be better able to grasp the need for treatment that's ongoing, though intermittent.

But what if she had asked me at the first visit: "I've already used a Class 6 steroid, Doctor, and it says right here on my online health program that the one you're giving me is just another Class 6 steroid. What is the basis for predicting that your steroid will be more efficacious than the ones which have failed?"

Good question. To answer it, I would have to admit that the cream isn't objectively stronger, but that she'll be more likely to stick with it because of my professional authority and calm reassurance. How would that go over?

Only she doesn't ask, not because she is uninterested or unintelligent, but because medical care is about more than patient autonomy and reportable outcomes. Among other things, it's about hope, fear, and trust.

I sometimes dream that every day I have to justify every clinical decision to a higher authority. Then I wake up, bathed in sweat and the relief that comes with realizing that I am no longer a raw trainee and still retain some clinical independence.

I cherish this independence. It is shrinking.

Dear Doctor, I'm the Specialist Your Patient's Hairdresser Recommended

Early in practice I got the feeling that other doctors made dermatology referrals with a different mindset than the one they used for referrals to other specialists. First meetings with patients often went something like this:

"Mrs. Flemm, I see by your sign-in form that Dr. Beech-Komber gave you my name."

"Not exactly."

"What do you mean?"

"When I told him my problem, he said, 'You'd better go see some skin man.' I actually got your name from my hairdresser. She says you're excellent."

Then came the proliferation of HMO's, with their requirements for referrals and rosters of approved doctors. These changes helped dermatologists like me develop the same intense personal relationships with referring physicians that we had with the Yellow Pages.

"Dr. Retro referred you, Mrs. Gidwitz?"

"No, but her secretary gave me three names from the Bay Colony Healthcare book."

Bound by old-fashioned etiquette, I wrote to thank the doctor anyway:

Dear Dr. Retro,

Thank you for referring Ernestine Gidwitz, who, as you know, has had dry skin for the past few decades. She gets relief from emollients and the coming of spring. Her rash suggests atopic eczema. I prescribed a cortisone cream. Her planned visit to Palm Springs should also help. Thank you for allowing me to participate in the care of this extraordinarily fascinating and pleasant patient.

With all good wishes.

I imagined this note prompting a puzzled exchange between doctor and receptionist:

"Harriet, Ernestine Gidwitz was here last week for her annual. Why did I get a letter from a dermatologist?"

"Remember, on her way out she said she's itchy?"

"Oh yeah, but who's this guy Rockoff?"

"We found him in the book. Ernestine says she knows his building because her manicurist is across the street."

Hoping to help doctors remember me, I began composing letters I hoped would make up in style what they may have lacked in riveting substance:

Dear Dr. Mudgeon,

Thank you for referring Mrs. Noonan, who, as you know, has many warts on her hands. Seeing her reminded me that four years ago you referred the Noonan twins, Rusty and Ricky, who also had many warts. After I froze one of Ricky's, he developed the most prodigious blood blister I've ever seen. Needling it to relieve pressure made it explode and spray reddish fluid all over my wallpaper. Thank you for helping me relive this moment in memory.

Fondly.

I considered another note a model of symmetry and concision:

Dear Dr. Schwab,

Thank you for referring Rabbi Hyatt. I removed the keratosis from his temple, so he could return to the Temple without his keratosis.

Cordially.

Some doctors responded with thanks for my helping relieve their staff's humdrum routine. I could only guess at what the ones who didn't respond were thinking.

Eventually, though, I had to rein in my expressiveness on advice of counsel. A plaintiff's lawyer sent me a threatening letter on behalf of a client who alleged that my diagnosis of neurotic excoriations was incorrect and that my misdiagnosis had resulted in permanent scarring. My malpractice insurer considered the claim meritless and had it dismissed. I was nevertheless disconcerted to find in her file the following referral letter:

Dear Terry,

Thank you for referring Glinda O'Shaughnessy. I did my best to reassure her that the lesions on her face are not "an infection I picked up in the Orient." We discussed the role of stress and ways to minimize it. Unfortunately, her plans to take a three-week trip around the world with her mother may not be the best way to start.

Gratefully,

The thought of hearing that read aloud in court dampened my enthusiasm for creative referral letters. Other doctors' receptionists would have to look elsewhere to relieve tedium.

Since then I stick to straightforward, boring notes, keeping running commentary unwritten. For instance (commentary in parentheses):

Dear Dr. Crabtree,

Thank you for sending over Mr. Chang Leung [or hiring someone with the good judgment to do it for you]. The cream you prescribed, though quite potent, has not cleared up his rash [because it's a fungus cream, and he doesn't have a fungus]. I also reassured him that the mole near his navel that you suggested he keep an eye on [and which he's been checking every six hours ever since] is benign and can be ignored until he sees you for his physical next year [his psychotherapy for hypervigilance should be well under way by then, anyway]. We also discussed the items on the list he brought [twelve miscellaneous "skin things" he's been saving up since puberty] for which I offered diagnoses [by translating his complaints into

Latin] and therapy [when available].

Again, thank you [or whomever] for referring this patient. [Send lots more!]

Gratuitously,

Alan Rockoff, MD

But Enough About You

"Study Says Chatty Doctors Forget Patients"
New York Times, June 26, 2007

"How are we today, Mr. Troldhaugen?"

"Well, Doctor, I have this itch. You know, down below..."

"Oh, don't I know it! I've been fighting that for years. Itch can drive you crazy. It's embarrassing too. I mean scratching in public is always awkward, but when you're a dermatologist...What have you been doing for it?"

"I have this fungus cream the druggist gave me."

"That figures. Fungus is usually the first thing everybody thinks of. I had the same experience last time I tried to treat myself. I have all these samples, so I tried one. It was hard to remember to put it on twice a day—made me more sympathetic when my patients don't always follow instructions exactly the way I give them. Anyhow, after a while it got pretty obvious that I was going to need something different, so I took a different sample and sure enough that did the trick."

"Maybe you can prescribe that for me…"

"It's interesting how common symptoms like these are. People I know often come over to me outside the office to ask pretty much the same questions, about itch and rashes and so forth. Of course, I can't exactly examine them there in the street or in their living rooms, but I can get a pretty good idea of what they have and what they need. After all, I've had the same symptoms myself…"

"So what would you recommend for me…?"

"And sometimes I've tried to share my experiences when I've had the same things as my patients do, just to show them that their situation isn't as strange or as frustrating as they might have thought. Take my wart, for instance…"

"But I don't have a wart."

"But I did—on my left thumb. Now that's interesting right there, because I'm right-handed. People always assume that warts are a contagious virus, but if they were—and I certainly shake hands with a lot of wart patients every day—why would they spread to my left thumb? But in any case it took me four years to get rid of mine, even though I have liquid nitrogen so I can freeze myself anytime I want, and I did too. So I used to tell that to people with resistant warts, so they wouldn't feel so frustrated."

"Doctor, about my skin problem…"

"And you know what? I found that people really didn't want to know about my problems, whether they were the same kind as theirs or not. In fact, patients weren't all that interested in what was going on with me in general. Of course, there are some people who've been seeing me for almost thirty years, who are old friends by now. They know the names of my grandchildren and ask after them, that sort of thing. But most other patients don't really want to know what I've been up to, where I'm going on vacation, or what staffing and administrative hassles I'm dealing with. Which kind of seems right, when you consider that they've come not to find out what's wrong with me but what's wrong with them. Doesn't that make sense?"

"Yes, but…"

"And then I read in the paper that they did this study in Rochester, with hidden mikes or something, and they found out that doctors were gabbing about their own weight problems and exercise programs, apparently with the thought that this would produce greater rapport. Instead, when the doctors heard tapes of what they said, they realized that maybe not 100 percent of the time, but most of the time talking about themselves had more to do with the doctors than with the patients. Can you believe that?"

"To tell the truth, I can…"

"It's just amazing how people can see faults in other people but not notice it in themselves. Isn't that right, Mr. Trondheim?"

"Troldhaugen."

"Right. Well, it's been nice chatting with you. Did I give you a prescription?"

Are You Sure?

The fear in Karen's eyes was obvious. I had just told her the moles she was worrying about looked normal. "Are you sure?" she asked.

Gently but firmly I replied, "Yes, I'm sure. I'll recheck them in a year, unless you bring a change to my attention before then."

"I know doctors hate when you ask that," said Karen, "but I had to."

Yes, we do hate when they ask that. The question, "Are you sure?" sounds reasonable enough, but in fact violates an unstated consensus and puts the professional relationship on a new and uncomfortable footing.

The usual understanding between patient and doctor is worth making explicit. The doctor says, "In this life, certainty is not possible, but I'll do the best I can and take special care to head off mistakes that can't be corrected." And the patient says, "Yes, I understand, and agree to accept your advice on those terms."

We all have a similar implicit consensus with the various people we rely on for advice and prediction, from mothers to friends to stockbrokers to weatherpersons, all the folks who tell us what to expect and how to deal with it. Do these advisors sometimes get it wrong? Sure. Do we stop asking them? Rarely. To err is human, we admit, and besides, we have to ask somebody.

Now suppose we changed the rules, and demanded from these advice-givers, "Are you sure?" What we would in fact be saying is, "Okay, buddy, I'm going to hold you to your prediction, and if it's wrong, I'm going to let you know what I think and take whatever action I deem appropriate." Such a change in the rules would have a chilling effect. Our advisors would think twice about opening their mouths, and might decide not to do so at all. Whether such reticence would leave us better off is another matter.

We all know how tough it is to care for other physicians and their families. We lose our "clinical instincts," and start ordering all kinds of tests we wouldn't bother with otherwise. The reason for this is that patients who are in the profession *always* ask, "Are you sure?" even if they never open their mouths. We fear that if we get it wrong, or even if things just don't turn out well, our colleagues will be less willing to cut us slack than the average patient would. And so we strive for certainty, even though that is no more attainable just because the patient happens to be a physician.

So what do we do when the patient is fearful, peremptory, or has an MD? With the challenge, "*Are you sure?*" ringing in our ears, we can:

- Say, "Yeah, pal, I *am* sure, and whaddaya gonna do about it?" This may work in the short term, but blow up in our faces if later events belie our bravado.

- Cave in and waffle. Humility is admirable in some settings, but acting uncertain does not inspire the assurance patients need to follow through on our recommendations.

- Find a middle ground, which implies confidence without arrogance. This can be subtle and tricky, especially when difficult people or circumstances put us on the spot. Choices may involve ordering tests or scheduling extra visits we hadn't contemplated. Compromise with dignity is a good strategy in a lot of situations, medical and otherwise.

I have one advanced technique for dealing with such situations, which I will describe without actually endorsing, because it's not for everyone. This consists of changing my opinion 180 degrees without admitting that's what I'm doing.

"Doctor, I'm worried about this mole!"

"The mole looks fine."

"Are you sure? Look, it's got a hair in it!"

"I think we should take it off right away, just to be sure."

If you've been around awhile, you won't be surprised to hear that this unacknowledged about-face rarely elicits a, "Hold on—you just said it was okay!" Instead, patients act relieved. "Great, Doc," they say. "Better safe than sorry!"

Of course, you have to keep a completely straight face all the way through for this technique to work. But it's neat when it does.

I'm sure!

Waiting Room Literature

"You play a lot of golf—right, Doc?"

"No, why do you ask?"

"You have *Golf* magazine in your waiting room."

"Have you got your own plane, Doc? I see you subscribe to *Flying*."

Actually, I subscribe to neither. Along with many other magazines, these rags come unbidden, like heartburn.

The waiting room of the GP we used as a kid had only ancient copies of *National Geographic*. I still recall their ugly yellow covers and stupefying articles. ("The Rat-Eaters of Borneo: A Mystical Journey.") Nowadays of course the periodicals our patients peruse while they wait reflect not just our personal choice but the pervasive blare of marketing, tie-ins, synergy, and all the rest of it. Bicyclists wear logos on their butts to tout energy bars, and doctors display mags to hawk everything from moisture lotion to made-for-TV movies. Some are magazines we've subscribed to, others just show up, leading patients to draw erroneous conclusions about our avocations and use of disposable income.

"Did your tomatoes come in good this summer, Doc? You get *Obsessive Gardener*."

"Where do you moor your yacht? You have *PersonalCruising* out there."

I visited my own waiting room to see which magazines we get.

People is one we actually want. A doctor's office is a great place to catch up on the celebrity gossip everybody wants to know about but nobody will admit reading. Given my own heavy load of medical journals, I myself have no time of course to keep up with Rob's comeback, Brad's wedding, or whether Britney's navel is collecting any lint.

In contrast, more substantive newsweeklies come to me all by themselves, sheathed in a glossy promo for eczema lifestyle suggestions or toenail fungus pills. Peeling off one of these recently revealed the cover story, "Who Needs a Husband?" illustrated by the cast of *Sex and the City*. Now *that's* hard news.

We also get a couple of women's magazines, some by subscription and others through spontaneous generation. These are a bit too popular, often disappearing within hours of arrival. Only the ones pitched at the twelve- to eighteen-year-old demographic hang around.) Women's magazines have pneumatic babes on the cover and a lineup of articles adhering to a rigid formula: a splashy lead on new advances in erotic technique ("Global Warming: Sex Tips from the Green Party"), followed by a piece on relationships, one on health, one on fashion and beauty, and a second piece on sex.

("Orgasm—New Horizons!")

Lately they've started sending us magazines for men that imitate traditional women's rags, just that models are beefy and articles cover what manly men presumably like to read about: sex ("Better Lovin': Which Supplements?"), fitness, and adventure ("I Bagged a Rabid Reindeer with a Swiss Army Knife.") Patients see those gleaming pecs and draw their own conclusions about what they can look like if they read what's inside.

"Say, Doc, you must pump a lot of iron."

All these periodicals print images that reinforce the stereotypes of beauty and fitness abroad in the land. Except for Cindy Crawford with her signature beauty mark, all men and women have flawless skin, no blemishes or moles of any kind, and both sexes' bodies are totally hairless. Those of us who perform laser hair removal appreciate this recent cultural preference.

There are also a few magazines like *Discovery* that print essays of general interest. I get a kick out of entering an examining room to find patients disappointed that they haven't had time to finish this really interesting article. I assure them that after their appointment they can stay in the waiting room for a while to finish reading. They never do.

Purveyors of subscriptions can be relentless. Last month a man called. "If you subscribe to one of our magazines," he said, "part of the proceeds go to support the Special Olympics."

"Skip the magazines," I said. "I'll donate to the Special Olympics directly."

He wouldn't hear of it, of course. Charity tie-ins, subscriptions, even the articles themselves, are window dressing for the ads and promotions in and on waiting-room magazines. Increasing visibility for these ads is what pays the caller's commission.

Though it's obviously not always possible, perhaps the best way to deal with material in the waiting room is to stay on time so patients won't have time to read any of it.

Good Doctors

I was flattered.

Vladimir had brought in his eczematous infant for a second opinion. No doubt he chose me because his GP was unsure, and he'd heard I'm boarded in pediatrics.

Not exactly.

In fact, he had already consulted a well-known academic pediatric dermatologist. "I was waiting for the commuter train in Sharon," said Vladimir. "I met this Russian guy and asked him if he knew a good dermatologist."

It's nice to hear that some Russian commuter thinks I'm good. But how does he know? And what is a good doctor, anyway?

This is not an idle question. Pay-for-performance is the Next Big Thing. Already insurers are rewarding hospitals for practicing "better medicine." Prodded by Medicare, professional associations are developing quality guidelines. Insurers have already started "tiering" doctors, hoping to steer patients with graded co-payments toward choosing "better, more efficient" doctors (as assessed by opaque and arcane formulas).

Fine, what's a better doctor?

This question is too complex for the likes of me to address in depth. I've observed, however, how hard it is to judge physician quality even when we want to, such as when referring patients to skin cancer surgeons, internists, ophthalmologists, allergists, and so forth.

When people are referred to me, they often say things like, "Dr. Smith says you're terrific!" Since I've only seen a handful of Dr. Smith's patients and have never met him, how does he know I'm terrific? Can he gauge my diagnostic acumen? Does he know my outcome data?

When I refer, I also say my colleague is swell; I want the patient to feel confident. Although I really believe the doctor is good, critical assessment forces me to concede that my evidence is thin. What, after all, do I really know about the doctor I'm referring to?

- Patients say his staff is nice.

- She sends prompt referral letters.

- He'll see an emergency right away.

- I once met her in the hall, and she seemed personable.

Such criteria imply something about my colleagues' character and managerial skills, but not much about competence. Is the internist a sharp diagnostician? Would she nail a rare tropical disease if it came her way? How would I know? Since the people I send her mostly need routine physicals, does it matter? I guess the skin surgery guy has good technique—he sends pictures of gaping wounds and neat stitching. But is he better or worse than anybody else? I have to admit I'm in no position to judge.

If doctors aren't too clever at recognizing quality, patients are worse. At times most of us learn about truly terrible physicians: they miss basic diagnoses, treat patients with casual contempt, do surgery beyond their ability, biopsy anything that moves. They're still in practice because most of their patients are still breathing. And many of these doctors have one striking thing in common:

They are wildly successful. Their patients swear by them.

And why not? Are laymen truly in a position to judge the competence of the professionals we consult or even the tradesmen we engage? How good a job does our accountant do? Our electrician? We may love them dearly right up to the IRS audit, or the fire from faulty wiring.

In other pursuits gauging quality may be fairly straightforward: gardening, auto repair, taxidermy. Defining excellence in medical care is harder, for reasons too numerous to list.

Soon, however, we're going to have to do it anyway, because those who pay our bills want value for their money. And they say value means "quality care."

So they've started with dramatic procedures with easily-measured outcomes, like mortality rates for transplants. For the rest of us, they want process data: how often doctors measure certain blood values in diabetics, prescribe steroid inhalers to asthmatics, and so on. Good process may turn out to produce good outcome, or it may not. Either way we're going to both do the right thing and—most crucial—report that we did it. If we don't, the counters of beans will be displeased, and our efforts won't count.

Will this make us better doctors? Consider: everyone agrees that a good doctor assesses whether patients who take the powerful acne drug Isotretinoin understand precautions. Before a prescription can be renewed, the federal online tracking program forces us to click the box, "In my opinion, this patient understands and is capable of complying with the requirements of this program." Does forcing us to click this box make us better?

For years we've struggled with HMO requirements for primary care referrals, occupational safety requirements, office laboratory setup demands. We've worked to fine-tune diagnostic and therapeutic codes and placate the alphabet soup of oversight agencies. All this highlights the futility of trying to resist the oncoming bureaucratic tide. Soon we'll have more boxes to click, along with online physician-quality tables for patients to peruse.

But many will still find their way to excellence the old-fashioned way.

Like Eddie, who has a rare and debilitating neuropathy that makes it almost impossible for him to walk. "I'm seeing Dr. Lariat over at St. Anselm's," he says.

"I hear he's tops," I reply. "How'd you find him?"

"Funny," says Eddie. "My brother-in-law Dave has box seats at Fenway Park—they're great, right behind third base. Turns out that guy in the next box is a neurologist at MBH. When Dave tells him what I've got, the guy says, 'Neuropathy? He's gotta see Lariat over at St. Anselm's. He's the best!'"

Dermatologic Drama

For many years I've sent starry-eyed youths off to New York or LA to seek their fortune on Broadway or in Hollywood. I wish them luck, asking only that when they win their Tony or Oscar they remember who cleared up their skin.

I'm still waiting.

If their goal is to write, I also ask that they pen a work starring a dermatologist. Medicine has been fertile ground for many gripping movie and TV dramas, but these seem to center on emergency rooms, charismatic neurosurgeons, or internists with character disorders. Not a skin doctor in the bunch.

The only TV show that paid much attention to our specialty was *Seinfeld*. Who can forget Jerry itching after removing his chest hair, Jerry finding a tube of antifungal cream in his girlfriend's medicine cabinet, or Jerry deriding a dermatologist date as "Doctor Pimple Popper," only to have an adjacent diner offer profound thanks for her lifesaving discovery of his melanoma?

So skin has had its moments. But however we hope that our specialty contributes to human happiness, we have to admit that the sometimes obsessive details of our daily work can play for laughs, not for pathos.

Nevertheless, I want to share the one episode in my career that did have real dramatic tension. If any reader wants to develop this incident into a TV pilot, please have your people call my people.

It happened this way:

One day a friend called to say that seventeen-year-old Melvin was in the hospital with infections in both armpits. Oral antibiotics having failed, his physician had admitted him for intravenous therapy, again with no results. The family suggested a dermatology consult, and the physician agreed. Would I come over?

Of course I would! I rarely visit hospitals anymore, but the opportunity to help out a family friend was welcome—especially since I was pretty sure I knew what her son had and what to do about it. I expected no direct communication from the attending physician, and got none. I finished work, drew up some injectable cortisone, packed alcohol pads and gauze, and headed over to the hospital.

There I found Melvin flanked at the bedside by his anxious mother and a family friend. Both were married to physicians, raising the stakes. They explained the situation: Melvin had an infection so severe that even intravenous antibiotics had failed. What could be done?

I asked whether Melvin ever had anything like this before. He had not. I examined him and found the expected.

I stood up and faced the family. In grave tones of reassurance and sagacity learned from reruns of *Masterpiece Theatre* I said, "Melvin does not have an infection. He has hidradenitis suppurativa." This sounded more like an incantation than a diagnosis.

"Is that serious?" asked the mother.

"It can be easily treated," I explained. "In fact, I brought the treatment with me."

"But this must be a serious infection!" said Melvin. "Even IV's aren't helping."

"They aren't helping," I replied evenly, "not because you have a serious infection but because *you have no infection at all.*"

(Swelling violins. Cut to station break.)

After some further discussion, I convinced Melvin, his mother, and her neighbor that cortisone injections into the armpit swellings were the right thing to do. I injected Melvin and promised to return the following morning. My satisfaction at hearing the family's thanks was tempered by anxiety. Was this exotic diagnosis with so many syllables correct? Would the treatment actually work?

When I entered Melvin's room early the next morning, I was met with smiles of profound relief and heartfelt gratitude. The swellings gone! The patient relieved! The unpronounceable presumption validated!

The transference in the room was thick enough to cut with a knife. I accepted the family's praise with becoming modesty, of course, but couldn't resist the thought: How truly neat. Sure diagnosis and prompt success at the hospital bedside—by a dermatologist!

(Clashing cymbals. Cut to scenes from next week's episode.)

Well, maybe there won't be an episode next week. Though I still savor the unique circumstances of this small drama, I must admit that some medical specialties are just not cut out for prime time. But at least we're not alone.

Can you imagine a TV miniseries, "PSA: Memphis, Forensic Urologists?"

Me either.

Curbside Consults

Cousin Maisie flew in from Akron with a juicy recurrent herpes cold sore on her lower lip. I advised an anti-herpes antibiotic. Her twelve-year-old Chloe had a scaly rash on her cheeks. Although Maisie said the pediatrician thought it was unusual, it seemed ordinary enough to me, so I suggested over-the-counter cortisone. Maisie's mom, Philomena, has many age spots on her face. "The dermatologist said she could take them off before Eunice's wedding," she complained, "but she'll charge $1,600."

I offered to do it for $1,590.

Three impromptu consultations at one family get-together. About average, I'd say.

Being asked medical advice outside the office is commonplace for all doctors, but perhaps more so for dermatologists, since skin questions are universal and symptoms mostly visible. Settings may vary; there is the traditional Curbside Consult for the commuter, the Dinner Party Consult for the gregarious, the Vestry Consult for the devout.

Most of my Vestry Consults take place in the synagogue: in the sanctuary, downstairs at the collation, or (in fine weather) on the street outside. An average Saturday is usually good for two or three. Last week, for instance, my friend the podiatrist showed me psoriasis on his hands, an older guy was worried about a benign thing on his face, a woman I hardly know asked me to look at a blood vessel on her daughter's face (the rotten kid buried her chin and howled, just like in the office). Thankfully, another dermatologist just joined our congregation. I love sharing opportunity with younger colleagues.

Vestry Consults are, of course, ecumenical. Last year Dot, an African-American woman with stasis dermatitis, asked me an endocrine question I thought should be directed to her gynecologist.

"I'll ask him in church this Sunday," she said.

"Dandy idea," I replied.

Some doctors complain that Curbside Consults are inappropriate and unfair. In general, I don't agree. Mostly, I find them harmless, even a bit flattering. People ask us because our profession has useful information to offer about things they wonder and worry about. If we can quickly and easily satisfy their wonder and allay their worry, why not?

It's human nature to walk around with questions you wouldn't make a professional appointment to answer, but would be sorely tempted to ask should the relevant expert suddenly materialize. Admit it: you see the auto repair guy on the street, the broker at a party, the sports celebrity in the mall. Don't tell me you *always* bite your tongue and suppress the urge to blurt, "My Mazda rattles on the freeway!" "When's the market turning around?" "How *about* those Red Sox?"

Most people apologize before asking us. "I know I shouldn't...," they stammer. "I hate doing this, but..." Then they do it anyway. Trying to stop them would be like interrupting a joke you've heard before. Reasonable enough, but it just embarrasses everybody.

Besides being apologetic before and grateful after, Curbside Consulters usually limit themselves to simple, answerable questions. Few bring up complicated or threatening issues that would involve lengthy discussions, or disrobing. When they do, a gentle suggestion that they call their own doctor or make an appointment usually meets with ready acceptance.

Not always, of course. There was the lady who started to hike up her skirt on the street to show me how her jock itch was doing. There was the guy who, at a charity event in a swanky hotel, joined me in a broom closet for a brief drawers-drop. When I run into him, we smile at the recollection of our small intimacy.

Medicine is about both helping people and making a living. Forcing people to ask questions only in our offices, insisting that helping and earning can't be separated, strikes me as a little mean-spirited. The sort of thing you'd expect from, say, a lawyer.

They tell of the doctor who complained to his attorney friend about consultations at curbside.

"The way I handle it," said the lawyer, "is I answer the question, then go back to the office and send them a bill."

"Great idea!" said the doctor. "That's what I'll do."

Two days later the doctor got a bill.

Was That You?

"Good morning, Mr. Nesia. I see you haven't been here in fifteen years."

"I was never here before."

"Forgive me—aren't you Alford M. Nesia, 36 Endive Gardens, Boxboro, date of birth, April 5, 1954?"

"Yes."

"In that case you were here in August of '91."

"I did see a dermatologist once, come to think of it. Was that you?"

It's always nice to know you've made a strong impression. Of course, forgetfulness works both ways:

"Nice to meet you, Ms. Jones."

"I saw you last month, Doctor."

Ouch. This usually happens when my staff checks in an old patient as a new one. Sometimes they haven't been able to find the patient's name in the computer (misspellings, data loss, a twenty-year absence, whatever). In other cases, the patient has come with a child or relative, but never registered as herself. I have a pretty good memory, but without a chart I'm mostly lost.

Unrecognized patients often make allowances: "You have so many patients, Doctor. You can't possibly remember them all." True enough.

I do try, though. People are often flattered when recognized, offended when they're not. (That's why politicians make such a point of remembering everyone.) Knowing who people are is a good start, but recollecting personal details is even better. I often note such details in the chart, whether or not they're germane to skin complaints. The patient may have started a new job, graduated college, bought a condo, planned a honeymoon in Uzbekistan.

When notes jog my memory about such things, I deftly slip in a personal reference while writing a prescription. "The Doxycycline is refillable three times, Ned. By the way, how *was* the bridal suite at the Samarkand Motel 6?"

If the patient exclaims, "You have a good memory! How did you remember that?" I usually confess that I'd written it down. That doesn't seem to offend anybody; instead they're somewhat pleased to have a stranger show some interest in their non-medical lives. I do it to make people comfortable and to get to know them a bit, since many of them come back at odd intervals over the course of many years.

I have another reason, too—a dark secret now revealed here for the first time: I occasionally find patients' stories even more riveting than the diagnostic and therapeutic challenges posed by their rashes and skin growths. There, I said it.

Outside the office, I'm even more lost when greeted by patients who recognize me. By now I've been around long enough that it's hard to go to the grocery or the gym or to just walk down the street without running into someone who stares, grins, and says, "Dr. Rockoff—is that you?"

I usually admit that it is and smile brightly in apparent recognition, keeping a keen eye out for an escape route before further conversation can unmask my ignorance of who the dickens they are. ("You know me! The one with the rash!") My father, well known in our hometown, was often hailed by strangers. He always smiled heartily and waved back. "Who was that?" I'd ask. "I have no idea," he'd say. "But they seem to know me, so I wave."

Of course, it's hard to recognize people out of context. I think my patients should have an easier time remembering me than I do them; after all, there are so many of them and just one of me. For the most part that's true, but some folks are just better at remembering than others.

"Nice to meet you, Mr. Steele."

"I met you already."

"Well actually, the one time you were here before you saw my associate Henrietta."

"You know, you're right—it was a lady!"

Glad we straightened that out.

You're Doing Great!

Aunt Bessie was beaming. She stopped by my office after her physical with her doctor up on the third floor. "I got a good report!" she exclaimed. "Dr. Wax was delighted with my x-ray, and she just couldn't get over how the swelling in my ankles has gone down."

You would think she was in grade school and had just gotten a great report card. In a way, you'd be right.

Years ago I read a book that attacked chiropractors as shameless, self-promoting hucksters. By way of evidence the author cited a pamphlet offering advice for new practitioners eager to build up their practices. Sample tip: Develop a repertoire of positive things to say. "You're doing very well today, Mrs. Jones," "Coming along nicely, Mr. Smith," and so on.

How tacky, I thought. Isn't telling the patient she's getting better just an indirect way of saying how terrific you are?

Well maybe, but not necessarily. And even so, it might be worthwhile anyway.

If patients were objective, they would view the course of their disease with clinical detachment. In that case they might assess the ups and downs of their symptoms the way they gauge the state of their neighbor's lawn. Green or weedy, facts are facts.

But patients are not objective. They view the course of their disease the way they look at the state of *their* lawn. Deterioration means more than distress or threat; it's a personal shortcoming—an embarrassing failure that reflects badly on them. It means they're coming up short, letting the side down. Letting *us* down. Doing well means the opposite.

Back in school if the teacher said, "Excellent answer, Sidney!" you glowed. If she frowned and shook her head, you felt rotten. You reacted this way even though hearing the teacher's opinion didn't make you one bit smarter or dumber. Patients react the same way even though the way we assess their progress doesn't make them any healthier or sicker. Like the schoolteacher, we're the authority in charge. Our opinion matters.

As such, it is perhaps better, when possible, not to be cool and objective but rather to praise a patient for doing well, as if he's achieved something special. Instead of giving you a funny look, he's likely to smile. He'll feel he's done a nice job by getting better. If told he's doing poorly, he'll react accordingly.

This is not a call for cynical spin, for making things up, pretending all is well when it's not, or for not trying to take appropriate steps to make patients do better than they have been. Even when things are not going as well as they might, there is always something positive to say.

- Your acne hasn't improved that much overall, but you don't have as many cysts as there were.

- Your psoriasis has a way to go but the plaques aren't as thick as they used to be.

- You do have another skin cancer, but it's very low-grade, and besides, you have fewer pre-cancerous sunspots than last time.

And so on. Whether or not this approach helps drum up business, it gives patients a hopeful outlook and makes them more likely to comply with the treatment plan. Beyond that, however, it just makes them feel better about themselves, their illness, and their general condition. It's worth recalling that patients visit us not just to reduce symptom scores, but to feel better.

Aunt Bessie's doctor obviously gets this. She sent a copy of Bessie's lab reports a few days later, extensively annotated in red pen to make clear which "abnormal" values were actually perfectly fine. In addition, the doctor had written this cheery assessment:

"Great labs, Bessie!"

This cheerleading tone may be a bit too bubbly for everyone's taste, but the impulse behind it is sound. Aunt Bessie beamed again.

My own internist clearly thinks the same way. Years ago he sent me a copy of my own laboratory tests, circled my cholesterol level, and wrote, "A-plus!"

I beamed from ear to ear. I was always a dutiful student, proud of my grades. Now I was proud of my cholesterol.

Verbal Boilerplate

There I was, lying on a gurney in a curtained compartment. Wearing a gown under a flimsy sheet and awaiting my five-year routine colonoscopy, I heard a doctor's voice from the next cubicle.

"Everything looked fine, Mrs. Jenkins," said the voice. "Just some small hemorrhoids. You might consider drinking a lot of water and eating a fiber-rich diet."

Although I'm no gastroenterologist, I know it when I hear it: verbal boilerplate. I even know it when I say it, though I try not to.

Boilerplate is a Victorian-age metaphor. From steel sheets that could be used over and over in different machines without change came the idea of reusable units of writing. No thought needed.

We all use verbal boilerplate every day, in and out of the office. ("How's everything?" "Fine." "What's happening?" "Not much.") Verbal boilerplate has two qualities: it's delivered without much inflection, and it doesn't convey a lot of information. The second quality can of course be useful. You don't *really* want to know how everything is, do you?

But in a professional context boilerplate has drawbacks. The way it's delivered signals what's really going on. That is how, although chilly and distracted, I sensed I was hearing boilerplate even before the words registered. The delivery was quieter, faster, flatter. Hemorrhoids? Press mental button: lotsofwaterfiberrichdiet.

The second aspect, not unrelated, is that verbal boilerplate is technically correct but doesn't say much. How much water is "lots?" How much fiber is "fiber-rich?" What kind of fiber? How often?

Maybe it doesn't really matter, but that's exactly the point: when you communicate with verbal boilerplate, what you're really saying is, "I'm telling you something I'm supposed to, but whether you understand or follow my advice isn't very important."

Such communication presents problems. The first is that from a medical standpoint, signaling that advice is not crucial is hardly a good way to promote adherence. (Reading studies about how often patients actually follow medical advice is always depressing anyway.) The second is that it's deflating to ask a serious personal question—which is how patients tend to think of their concerns—and get what amounts to a canned response.

We don't like to think we dispense boilerplate, but it can be hard not to. Talking to a new acne patient, how many novel and creative ways are there to present the basic spiel? No it's not food, yes you can use makeup, please don't pick your pimples, apply the creams and take your pills regularly, don't be discouraged if you don't clear up in two weeks, yada yada yada.

The same is true for eczema, warts, or any of the routine things any skin physician deals with daily. How tempting to succumb and dispense boilerplate: You've got disease X? Here is response Y. Gotta go now.

But avoiding this is possible without a lot of effort or time. The first step is to recognize the problem and listen to ourselves talk as though we're the patient. The second is to vary the mode of presentation, even if just a bit, between one visit and the next (by changing sentence order, or modifying phrasing). The third is to add emphasis to show we're making a point we really want to put across, and that it does matter whether the patient understands the instructions and knows how to follow the directions. The fourth is to maintain eye contact and vary inflection, to show that we are not automated attendants dispensing recorded announcements with implied or explicit disclaimers that the opinions herein expressed are not those of the management, the medical society, or the Department of Homeland Security.

Written boilerplate in a contract or lease agreement has lots of words in tiny print, to signal that you don't have to spend time reading it. Verbal boilerplate sends a similar message: careful listening isn't important. But in that case, why bother saying it?

A week after my gurney epiphany I got a letter from the gastroenterologist telling me I don't need another colonoscopy for five years. Now *that's* what I call meaningful communication.

The Doctor Will See You Later

I gave my name at the front desk of my new eye doctor. "Check in around the corner," said the clerk.

Two front desks, apparently. The secretary at the second one handed me some pages of demographics and medical history to fill out. In the meantime, she chatted with her associates as she scanned my insurance card.

I sat in the waiting room as instructed. After a short while a young man called my name. Since the ophthalmologist is a middle-aged woman, I realized at once that he was someone else.

"Hi, I'm Jeff," he said cheerily, ushering me into an exam room where he started to test my vision. ("What's the lowest line you can read? What's clearer—1 or 2? 3 or 4?")

After a few minutes, I softened my voice and said, "Please don't be offended. But who are you?"

"I'm Jeff," he explained.

"Yes, but what is your role here, exactly?"

"I'm an ophthalmic technician," he said. "The doctor will see you when I'm done examining you and dilating your pupils."

He proceeded. In our time together, I learned a few things about Jeff. (I'm nosy that way.) Being an ophthalmic tech was his second career. His first was building custom furniture, "until I blew out my shoulder helping a buddy on a weekend." Jeff's first eye job was in the cornea department of a teaching hospital, until slow business there limited his advancement options. So far he liked private practice. He tapped clinical data onto the computer screen to his left.

I returned to the waiting room. Shortly I heard my name again and through a dilated blur recognized the doctor herself. Her examination was businesslike, punctuated by more taps of data onto the screen. "You have early cataracts," she said. "Not clinically significant yet, but there." She said I didn't need new glasses unless I wanted a different style. "See you in a year," she said, exiting. I made that appointment at the first front desk.

There are many aspects of our practice world that shape what we do into a good or service, like building a cabinet or installing a dryer. There are codes for diagnosis and procedure; these generate a fee. There are measures of efficiency and outcome, which aim to streamline medical services, make them uniform, and lately to rate those who provide them. Much power and money are at stake, not to mention quality, now being energetically defined by the bureaucratic powers that be.

It's therefore understandable that for these and other reasons many doctors delegate history-taking to medical assistants, then counseling to other personnel. The doctor just comes in for the core service, the part that supposedly counts.

This seems a shame, for reasons I think go beyond sentiment, though maybe I'm fooling myself. (Without knowing the patient's background, level of motivation, and attitude toward the recommended regimen, how do you know he or she will follow it?) But larger forces outweigh objections like these. Anyhow, in my own small clinical domain I can still choose to learn some personal things about my patients, and act as though they matter. After all, I've known many of them for a long time, some for decades.

My own internist of twenty-five years limited his panel and joined a national concierge firm. (Concierge, or boutique, medicine means you pay a couple of grand a year on top of what your insurance does, for which you're promised quick appointments and the return of your calls.) A colleague upstairs agreed to take me on despite a closed practice.

Stan, in practice since the mid-1970s, is one of only three physicians who's been in my building longer than I have. He is quite a throwback. He has a small office, one secretary, and takes the medical history himself (no forms). He even does his own EKG's, if you can believe it. But he does use e-mail, and responds promptly.

You get the pleasant feeling that Stan actually knows who his patients are. This suggests that when the need arises, he doesn't just send his patients (and won't send me) off to a clutch of hospitalists and specialists to await their summary reports.

Stan is a vigorous guy, and he looks to practice another five years. Once he hangs 'em up, I may go with a concierge of my own. Sometimes when you want intimacy, or its illusion, you just have to pay for it.

Is It Cancer Yet?

It took me a while to catch on.

My first hint came at a free skin cancer screening years ago at our City Hall. I noticed that not all the patients who came were uninsured with no medical access. Many had dermatologists. Many had me.

"What about this dark spot, Doctor?"

"It's a seborrheic keratosis, Mrs. Jacobs. Comes with age. Completely benign."

"That's what you said at my last visit. I just wanted to see if it's still okay."

Fast forward to last Thursday. Dale is worried about some spots on her face.

"The ones on your chin are keratoses," I explain. "They're fine. And the flat ones on your cheeks are also no problem. If they don't bother you, they can stay."

Dale expresses relief. We chat for a few minutes, catch up on things. Then her eyes narrow. "Ah, tell me, Doctor…these spots could never become…cancerous, could they?"

Patients look at moles and spots in ways that are fundamentally different from the way doctors do. Simply put, to a medical professional a lesion is either benign or malignant. To a patient a spot is either malignant, or *not yet malignant*.

Perhaps we're suspicious about a lesion and perform a biopsy. The biopsy is benign. We delightedly report the good news. The patient is happy too, but just provisionally. Sure it's not cancer—today. Tomorrow, who knows?

Of course even in our scheme, benign moles can sometimes turn cancerous once in a very great while, but that uncommon transformation is not what worries patients. After all, every day we see moles that never, ever turn bad, which can't do so even in theory—because they lack the types of cells that can transform. For our patients, however, even these are potential malefactors who got off on a technicality. Better be vigilant; they could be back, armed and dangerous.

The difference between the way we look at things and the way our patients do is the difference between a thing and a process. To us a lesion is a collection of different kinds of cells. Each collection has an identity and an expected biologic fate. We look at all diseases that way too, and call them "entities." They have an independent existence outside the individual who has them. They behave in a certain way and respond to a variety of treatment methods.

To patients, a lesion is not a thing in itself but rather part of a process, specifically a deviation from what used to be, a signal of instability. The skin used to be clear; now there's something there. Something is going on. Once that starts to happen, who's to say it won't keep happening, leading finally to the ultimate instability: cancer.

No need to take my word for any of this. Watch and listen to a patient worried about a spot:

"We call this a dermal nevus, Mr. Perkins. It's completely benign"— Pause for effect—"and it will *always* be benign."

Mr. Perkin's eyes widen in surprise. This is indeed news to him. "You mean it will *always* be nothing to worry about? I had no idea…"

The conversation proceeds to other matters. Then, as he is about to depart, Mr. Perkins asks, "So this mole—it can never turn into cancer, right?"

No, he is neither deaf, nor hostile, nor linguistically or culturally challenged. The words he's been told are clear, but the concept they convey is so different from what he's always thought that its implications are hard to credit.

Of course, some people are more anxious about instability than others. If they—or the spouse who encouraged them to come to the office—are simply beyond reassurance, it may be best to just take off the offending spot so everyone can relax.

Suggesting that patients "keep an eye" on something is often unhelpful, if not counterproductive. Saying that implies that there is something to keep an eye on. If that's really so, the doctor ought to be the one to do the looking, or perhaps better, to remove it. It makes little sense to wait until *after* something turns cancerous to remove it.

Heaven help us if we had to take off every mole "just to be safe." Better to say, at least most of the time, that the spot in question is benign…and (guess what!) will *always* be benign.

Shedding a Tier

"Good news," says Stella the pharmaceutical rep as she unloads her samples. "Our Class IV steroid, Esterhazicort, is now Tier II on Babsoncare. That means patients have a co-pay of only $25."

Where do they get these names, I wonder. Hungarian focus groups? "How about the other insurers?"

"Still Tier III, $50 co-pay. But you don't have to fill out a pre-authorization form to get permission to prescribe it."

"Good."

"Remember," says Stella, "it comes in 15, 29.7, 43, and 122 grams. More size versatility than any other Tier III."

An unfamiliar face appears. "I'm Dick," he says, "with State Pharm. SulfacetaPOW is now Tier I with all Red Hook-managed care products. Just a $10 co-pay!"

"I thought Fritzi from Integumentum was the rep for SulfacetaPOW."

"We bought the brand from Integumentum," says Dick, "for cash, future considerations, and Dutch McGriff."

"Who's Dutch McGriff?"

"Left-field prospect for Double-A Topeka. Good arm, hits to all fields."

"How about Babsoncare?"

"Still Tier II," he says. "Same with Brandeis-Puritan. VesuviusHealth is Tier III. But there's no pre-authorization needed, and we have rebate coupons for the high co-pays. Where shall I put 'em?"

"In the closet, please, next to the other rebate coupons, special promotions, and limited warranties."

"Thanks. And don't forget that our product comes in eighty-four ounce jugs, so it's more economical for your patients."

I am having trouble storing this data in my aging parietal lobes, especially since the data keeps changing. So many insurers, so many new drugs, so many Tiers.

All this memorization is giving me a headache, so I see my neurologist. It's a migraine, he says, and gives me a bag of twelve samples—four each of different classes of medications. He tells me to pick one that works. Three of them do. I call my pharmacist.

"You have my insurance information in your computer," I say. "I've got SHPILCA, through my wife. Can you tell me which of these is low-tier on SHPILCA?"

"No, I can't," says the pharmacist. "First you have to hand us a prescription. Then we can put it through to find out how it's covered."

My head pounds. The hospital's PHO (or is it SUV?) is threatening that if I don't meet my quota of 87.2 percent generic scripts, they will take unspecified but unpleasant action.

In walks Stan. "Fabulous news," he says. "Our new product Fungiscram works by a new mechanism—it insults funguses until they leave."

"What Tier?" I ask wearily.

"Tier 1 on Red Hook!" he exclaims. "Tier II on Vesuvius and Brandeis-Puritan. With Babsoncare we're Tier IV."

"I thought it only went up to III. What's Tier IV?"

"They confiscate your drug card and send you to the countryside for fiscal reeducation. But we do have a special offer—buy three tubes and get a Fungiscram tote bag."

"Into the closet, please."

I try to digest all this. Estherhazicort is Tier II on Red Hook, SulfacetaPOW is Tier I on Vesuvius...No, wait, that was Fungiscram. But the patient gets the co-pay back on the antifungal with Brandeis-Puritan...or was that the steroid on SHPILCA. No, I'm the one with SHPILCA, no one else has that. Or maybe it was the tote bag—no, the sunscreen. Hold on, it was Tier III with the larger container and the Disney World tie-in. But that was only Babsoncare if you qualified for the FrequentFarma discount...No, that's not right either. It was Tier III if you get the small tube and

Tier II if you get the bigger one...No, wait...

I slump down and sigh. The SUV will have my head. My brain isn't growing any more neurons. What will I say when they ask me, "Why won't you consider this effective and elegant product if it costs only a little more to your patient than generic and it comes in a larger container and there's a rebate coupon?"

I will have to throw myself on the mercy of the court:

"Please forgive me, but I CAN'T REMEMBER all the permutations of Tier and tube size and insurer and rebate. I have enough trouble making a diagnosis and prescribing treatment. Plus I have an excuse—I was trying to stuff six new biologic agents for psoriasis into my cortex. Also, I have this terrible headache, and the migraine drug I picked turned out to be non-formulary Tier III!"

I wonder if Dutch McGriff ever gets rashes.

Public Health

I'm not sure why I agreed to speak at the mall, and gratis at that. Maybe it was nostalgia for the talks I gave starting out thirty years ago to community groups, primary doctors, or TV interviewers at small, public-access stations. Or maybe I just like to talk.

When I got to the Waterville Mall at 9:45, my hopes for a good crowd rose when I saw lines of people stretching out into the lobby. That lasted until I realized they were there for the Registry of Motor Vehicles. My talk would be next door, at the Old Tyme Buffet. Posters announced this month's installment of the Health Awareness series, "Advances in Skin Cancer." I met Janice, a twenty-something in charge of marketing for the strip mall. She led me inside the still-closed restaurant.

"Usually, they're done vacuuming before the lectures start," she said. "You'll be speaking from here." She pointed to a blond-wood busing station against the near wall. I turned to face long, neat rows of small tables, each set with salt, pepper, ketchup, and steak sauce.

"How did you get my name?" I asked Janice.

"Google," she replied. "Would you believe we called thirty dermatologists before we found you? The others were too busy or not interested."

That was gratifying. "Do you get the same people coming to the lectures every month?"

"Pretty much," she said, indicating a list of regulars. "They check off their names so we can send them announcements."

By then people started showing up. They all seemed to know Janice and each other. "These are good seats," said one woman to her companion, taking a table in front.

Others shuffled in. By just after ten o'clock, fifteen people had signed in and sat down. All were old and wan. There were two men, one a stocky fellow with a trucker's cap and a T-shirt that read, "This is America. Please speak English." Janice handed out bottled water.

One woman sported a bulky gauze dressing on her left cheek. "My dermatologist took off a skin cancer this week," she said, heading to her table.

"What kind of cancer was it?" I asked.

"I don't know," she said. "I forgot to ask him."

Janice offered no introduction. She distributed my one-page handout.

As instructed, I had brought no slides or PowerPoint presentations; the restaurant walls were unsuitable for either. My sheet listed websites on which to find skin cancer pictures, though this crowd seemed unlikely to spend much time online.

I told them about basal and squamous cells, about melanoma, about UVA sunblocks and UVB sunblocks, about whether sun protection lowers your level of vitamin D. I criticized tanning parlors, and we shared chuckles about the foolishness of kids.

One woman rose to testify. "I know my skin cancer came from a terrible sunburn on my chest," she said. "My skin turned blue. Then I got this small, dark spot. One doctor said to forget about it, but I went to another one, and they did a test."

I agreed that sunburns are undesirable, but suggested that a single bad one wouldn't necessarily generate cancer.

"What strength sunscreen do you recommend?" asked one woman.

"He already answered that," said her tablemate. "You have to pay attention!" I assumed this pair shared similar interchanges every month.

And so it went. The props were different from those in the old days: instead of screens, slide projectors, or TV cameras, I now faced rows of inverted Heinz bottles. But the rest was familiar: the same facts, advice, questions, even my jokes and their predictable responses. Everything about those talks came flooding back, including why I'd stopped giving them.

The public can't get enough medical news. What they really want to hear about are breakthroughs and exciting advances. Those of us who don't live on the clinical cutting edge have more mundane fare to offer, less like what comes from the lab bench or operating suite than what emanates from the pulpit. Like pastors, we offer sage wisdom and sensible advice to people inclined to listen to us. They nod in agreement, and not much changes.

Also like pastors, we don't give up. The same regulars come time after time, only maybe this time they'll pay closer attention so that our words hit home and nudge them a bit in the right direction.

So maybe that's why I agreed to speak.

Or maybe I just like to talk.

Stop Me Before I Pun Again

People who call puns the most debased form of humor are just jealous. For the true aficionado, hearing groans of pain and watching eyes flash with threatened vengeance makes it all worthwhile. Why apologize? We are not punitent.

In a doctor's office, humor, debased or otherwise, should be used with discretion. Dermatology, however, where signs and symptoms are so deliciously concrete, often presents punning temptations too hard for mere mortals to resist. The flesh, so to speak, is weak.

How, for instance, can you keep from addressing baldness off the top of your head? If the lobe's been pierced, shouldn't you play it by ear? If the patient has an eyelid cyst, needn't we keep an eye on it? Isn't treating skin tags a pain in the neck? Why wouldn't an acne sufferer meet his problem head on and face up to it? Mustn't we stop eczema before it gets out of hand? Isn't Novocain worth a shot? Shouldn't the caring physician who pares a plantar wart peer into the patient's sole? Can he do so without being callous? Corny? So what if we sometimes give in to our weaker impulses—don't we accept our patients as they are, warts and all?

Trying to recall every punning opportunity would be rash. Even a long list would only scratch the surface, and why pick over old scabs? Still, it is hard to resist looking back from a ripe perspective at all the golden opportunities that got away, along with the ones that should have.

There was the psoriatic who hadn't been around in a while and was worried because his knee was newly affected. Was I wrong to observe that his knee, like himself, was a site for psoriasis? Was I callous to suggest that a patient anxious about a cyst on the skin above her spine just put it behind her? Or reassure her that I had her back? I keep many patients in stitches, some for ten days.

Sometimes punning is unintentional, at least consciously. A member of a traveling acting troupe once consulted me about a painful peri-anal rash for which a doctor in another city had prescribed a cortisone ointment. The patient lay prone on the examination table, flanked by a medical student on one side and me on the other, each of us peering into the cleft between a rather fleshy pair of buttocks. Finding a yeast colony thriving on their steroid-enriched diet, I started explaining to the patient that a different kind of cream would help. Not wishing to make myself look wise at the expense of his former physician, however, I added that it helped me to know the steroid cream hadn't worked. With mounting horror I then heard myself say, "Of course, I have the benefit of hindsight..." In the dead silence that followed, I added weakly, "If you'll pardon the expression." At that point all three of us lost our composure. I had to leave the room before regaining mine. Fortunately, the patient was a cheerful fellow who didn't seem to take offense.

But not every pun is unconscious. I recall the time that a patient of Finnish ancestry, who grew skin cancers like potatoes, brought his fiancée in to be checked. She, too, had been diagnosed with a basal cell carcinoma or two, and she wanted me to look at a tiny lesion on the rim of her left nostril.

Peering through a magnifying loupe with bright light at close range, I could barely make it out. "Looks okay," I said. "I can hardly see it."

"Please test it," she said. "The doctors also thought my last bump was benign, until they took a biopsy."

I looked again. "But I really can't see it," I said.

"Look, Doctor," she said, "I trust you and I appreciate your judgment, but it would really help my peace of mind if you tested it so I'll know for sure."

It was then that I experienced what can only be called a Punster's Epiphany: a sense of being controlled by a power larger than myself, a setup so perfect, circumstances so unique and unrepeatable, that failure to capitalize on them would mean an eternity of bitter punning remorse.

"Okay," I said, drawing a deep breath and focusing on keeping my voice steady and my face straight. "After all," I said, "it's no skin off my nose."

Though I deserved worse, the patient did not clobber me. And like my intentions, her biopsy was benign.

Community Outreach

"Hospitals Begin to Move into Supermarkets," *New York Times, May 11, 2009*

"The Cleveland Clinic has lent its name and backup services to a string of CVS drugstore clinics in northeastern Ohio. And the Mayo Clinic is in the game, operating one Express Care clinic at a supermarket in Rochester, Minnesota…

New York Times, May 11, 2009

"How may I help you?"

"I need frozen peas, strawberry jam, and a skin cancer screen."

"Frozen peas, aisle 6; jams and preserves, aisle 8; skin screens right here."

"Right here? Terrific."

"Yes, please undress and we'll have a look."

"In the aisle?"

"Just kidding. See the booth over there? Next to the deli counter.

Have you seen a dermatologist lately?"

"Yes, I got a screen at CostCutter last month."

"Then why do you need another one?"

"I just finished a tanning series to get ready for a cruise, and I'm feeling guilty and vulnerable. Do you offer other services besides screens?"

"Sure, what else have you got?"

"I have this wart on my index finger—OUCH! What was that?"

"Liquid nitrogen. What else is going on?"

"I've been breaking out."

"Skin cleansers, aisle 12; makeup, aisle 13. And here's a prescription."

"Thanks. Can I fill it anywhere?"

"We have an exclusive with OldMacDonald's Pharma. Anything else?"

"My wife gave me a list. Let's see, laundry detergent, Ovaltine, whole wheat muffins—oh, yes, she wants you to look at this mole on my scalp. HEY, CUT THAT OUT!"

"I just did a shave biopsy. We'll mail you the test results next week with our next batch of coupons. Please take this card."

"What is it?"

"Log onto our website and enter this eight-digit alphanumeric code. It makes you a member of our SuperShopper VIP Club, which entitles you to an emergency appointment at any one of our offices in under six weeks."

"Well, I guess all I need is that skin screen."

"Before you get undressed, would you like e-mail updates about our specials?"

"No thanks."

"In that case, I'll tell you about them now. Refer a friend or family member and get fifteen percent off any three products in our signature, private-label skincare line?"

"Okay, I'll see."

"Removal of brown age spots, half price?"

"No thanks."

"Laser off two blood vessels, get the third one free?"

"Not interested."

"Photorejuvenation, package of three, twenty percent off?"

"No, thank you. Wait, I just remembered that my wife needs help with a coleslaw recipe using low-fat mayo."

"Mayo clinic, aisle 3. Cleveland Clinic, aisle 2. Well, thanks for coming."

"Hold on, what about my skin screen?"

"Sorry, I forgot. Why did you want another one?"

"I'm tanned, guilty, and vulnerable."

"Right. In that case you should see my colleague."

"What colleague?"

"Psychiatrist. He's in fresh produce, behind the broccoli. Next!"

Body and Mind

A medical journal article published a few years ago found a "strong negative association...between psychiatric morbidity and compliance." (In other words, patients with psychiatric issues were less likely to follow treatment instructions.) The fact that such morbidity "was the strongest predictor of poor compliance" spurred the authors to urge..."timely identification and appropriate management of anxiety disorders and depressive disorders in everyday dermatologic practice."

As an everyday practicing dermatologist, I question that recommendation. What it says is that I should see to it that patients with anxiety and depression take care of those conditions. Of course I agree they should. It's just that I can't make them do it.

Psychological issues are important in daily patient management, often outweighing the physical ones. The problem is calling these issues what they are. In my own experience, patients who visit doctors who address disorders of the body don't want to hear that their problems have anything to do with their mind.

It doesn't take medical students on elective in my office more than two days to say, "This isn't dermatology—it's psychology!" Indeed. It takes as much time to help people ignore their symptoms as to make the symptoms go away. The key thing is to ferret out what's eating people (fear of cancer, contagion, decline) and explain why they can stop worrying. If they pick at themselves, I give them something else to do, perhaps a cream to apply. If fear of bugs or sun damage makes a patch of their skin tingle, I advise a topical anesthetic. If they're sure they're going bald when they aren't, I suggest a vitamin supplement, so they can stop paying attention to daily hair loss.

What I don't do very often is get explicitly psychological. People don't like to hear that their problem is anything but purely physical, and they make their displeasure clear. I hate being glared or yelled at. It's a psychic thing with me.

Yet because I am not too old to change, I attended a seminar on psychiatric management at the national dermatology meeting one year with an open mind.

The session leader seemed like a sensible, down-to-earth guy. He claimed that since there are good medicines to combat picking, we dermatologists should prescribe them. He suggested one pill in particular, an antidepressant that also fights picking behavior.

My friend Dan, a psychiatrist specializing in obsessive-compulsive disorder, has suggested that I familiarize myself with this class of drugs, since many patients I tell him about clearly are at least borderline obsessive-compulsives.

Okay, why not? The next time I saw patients with chronic picking,

I gave it a shot. Jennifer was scratching her face. Stanley had been picking all over for more than forty years. Neither seemed otherwise unbalanced, and each expressed willingness to try anti-picking medication, which I carefully explained worked by physical-chemical means (to limit psychiatric stigma).

I never saw or heard from either one again.

At times I see patients who do have major psychiatric problems. There was Douglas, for instance, who showered several times a day because he was convinced that semen might get on his hands and impregnate his girlfriend. He agreed he needed help. I referred him to Dan. He never went.

In fact, not one of the patients with frank obsessive-compulsive disorder I've sent to Dan ever consulted him. Or anyone.

I've gained further insight in this area from inquiries sent to me on the Internet. Many questioners have clear-cut psychological issues. One needn't be Freud to recognize this when someone writes that they haven't had sex in twenty years because of the white bumps on their genitals that their doctors diagnosed as normal cysts.

The impersonality of cyberspace lets me be forthright. "Get counseling so you can accept your body," I advise.

But this same impersonality allows the patient to respond with the kind of explicit aggression an office setting might inhibit. "How dare you belittle my symptoms with your psychological garbage?" responds the questioner.

You could, of course, argue that I just don't do a good job, that I unintentionally sabotage the psychiatric interpretation or referral.

All I can answer is that my best efforts over many years continue to convince me otherwise. People who see body doctors want body explanations. That we're aware of psychological dimensions may not lead to either effective management or appropriate referral.

And if psychiatric issues produce noncompliance, there may be little we can do, other than pretending to address the body with the true aim of mending the mind.

Bad Reviews

"Who gave you my name?"

"The Internet. I read your reviews."

More and more patients say things like this. So I Googled my reviews. Here's one:

This guy gave me a 5 min appointment. He did not listen to anything I had to say. I recommend NOT going to see him. Absolutely awful. Please please don't waste your money.

Maybe you're thinking: "It's cranky people who vent online. I'm sure Rockoff probably doesn't blow people off like that." If so, you are kind. Thanks.

But how do you really know? Maybe I do ignore what patients have to say. Or maybe I usually don't but did this time. Here's another review:

This doctor was a total waste of time. I go in and explain my problem, explain my pains. He proceeds to tell me that it is all in my head, and the pain is because I am thinking up having pain. REALLY? I spend my time trying to imagine pain? Please PLEASE do not go to ...

I like to think I counsel more sensitively than that, but maybe I didn't at this visit. Since the review is anonymous, I really don't know.

Online reviews are a fact of life. Authors I know ask their friends to plug their work on Amazon. I chose a beard trimmer based on an Internet review. (I hate the trimmer but don't have the time, or the bile, to share this with the hirsute universe.) When it comes to doctor reviews, legal experts tell us that we lack recourse to address egregious, even libelous, attacks on our professional competence, including those that could threaten our reputation and livelihood. Anonymity makes attacking easy and painless—to the attacker.

The 3 times I went he rushed the appointment, told me the wrong information regarding my skin problem, and was visible [sic] upset when I tried to ask questions to understand what was wrong with my skin which if he explained it properly ....

That isn't how I think I interact with people, but maybe I'm wrong. After all, offensive people don't know they're obnoxious. Perhaps this patient and I just didn't hit it off. If you deal with lots of people, some of them won't like you. Nothing new there.

But in the old days, dissatisfied patients just complained to a few friends and asked for their records. Now they can vent their spleen and post it to all humanity.

I think most doctors are ingratiating sorts. Unlike litigating attorneys or meter maids, we generally want people to like us. Even if we know not everyone will, it bothers us when they don't. We sometimes give a passing thought to the way we'll be remembered, to the extent that we are. We may hope that people will recall us as someone who cared and tried to help, even if we sometimes fell short, or failed.

Online reviews ensure that critiques of these failures, justified or not, become an enduring part of the public record. Imagine if this were true of personal relationships: if every relative we riled up, every friend we let down, every neighbor we crossed, didn't have to write a tell-all memoir (who would read it?), but instead could spend five delicious minutes getting even by assassinating our character for the whole world for all time. And anonymously—what bliss!

Online reviews are not going away, so whining about them is about as useful as complaining that air has too much nitrogen. One helpful strategy is to actively solicit positive reviews. This goes against my grain, but you have to move with the times. Happy patients will gladly post comments—if you ask them. I did this last week. Here's the review:

At a recent visit, I left waiting to hear back for results from a biopsy. Upon leaving, albeit a bit nervous, I thought about how assured I feel every time I meet with Doctor Rockoff. I know if I have to hear something dreadful, I would prefer to hear it from him.

Nice, yes? I may be Doctor Doom, but I do it with a smile.

Of course, the other reviews will remain, diluted but unexpunged. Oh, well. Keeps you honest anyway.

Rumors of My Death Have Been Greatly Exaggerated

"How did you get my name?" I asked.

"My sister came here ten years ago," she said. "She used to be a patient of Dr. Alvin Sherwin."

"I took over Dr. Sherwin's practice when he moved to Florida," I told her. "That was in 1981, so it's closer to thirty years ago, not ten."

"My goodness," she said. "That explains what my sister said."

"What did your sister say?"

"Well, my mother found your name on a piece of paper. My mother likes to hold on to things."

"I'll say she does," I said.

"She said, 'Why don't you call this guy Rockoff? He took care of your sister. He's very good.' So I looked you up and found your office.

"Anyway," she continued, "when I told my sister that I found you, she said, 'Yes, I remember seeing him. You mean he's still around? After all these years I figured he was probably dead.'"

"Well," I said, "not yet."

Who Will Take Care of the Patients?

My last medical student confirmed it: dermatology is one white-hot field. Only the very brightest dare apply, she told me, and even star students face long odds. One of her top classmates who failed to match for a position as a dermatology resident took a year off to do the research he needed to buff his resume.

A column I once wrote describing my experience hiring, training, and working with a physician assistant drew some strenuous responses from my colleagues. A few of these accused dermatologists like me who engage so-called physician extenders (physician assistants, nurse practitioners) of irresponsible venality.

When my physician assistant gave unexpected notice one year, I considered taking on a graduating dermatology resident. Directors at nearby training programs agreed to post my opportunity, but said they weren't sure how many in their graduating cohort actually planned to enter practice. I got no bites.

Shortly after that I spoke with a consultant, who shared some statistics, which I quote without being able to vouch for. He said the number of trainees sitting for the dermatology boards each year roughly approximates the number of practitioners who retire, but residents intending to practice are in fact much fewer. The rest, he said, "are interested in laser and skin surgery."

Later in the year I had a chance to confirm these comments, if only anecdotally. Interviewing two men about to finish their training, I learned that several of their fellow residents were indeed heading for careers other than general dermatology practice: cosmetic or surgery fellowships, or leaves of absence for family reasons.

A recent president of the American Academy of Dermatology noted with pride our specialty's popularity among students, adding, "Is it any wonder that our training programs are choosing from among the best and the brightest that medicine has to offer?" Such candidates, he adds, "include people who have founded their own companies, others who hold doctorate degrees as well as medical degrees, and top research scientists."

Attracting such applicants is indeed cause for pride, as well as optimism that a new generation of this caliber may make discoveries that will enhance our profession and benefit patients and society at large. A small doubt, however, nags.

Caring for patients with everyday conditions offers many rewards and demands special skills, but high-octane intellect and entrepreneurial moxie are perhaps not among them. If I am a super-bright young dermatologist with research credentials and interest, how will I view the banal task of managing acne, warts, and eczema? Will I approach it with relish, or consider it at best a necessary but annoying inconvenience?

Several trends, therefore, seem to point to this problem: if trainees see dermatology as an avenue to do exciting research, learn sophisticated technical skills, or advance lucrative cosmetic careers, then who will take care of the patients, the ones with common skin problems?

This is not a rhetorical question. In other countries dermatologists function as secondary or even tertiary consultants. You can't get to them unless you've been seen and treated first by primary or general practitioners. In principle, there is no reason that internists, family physicians, and pediatricians shouldn't manage basic skin problems in the United States as well, but those of us who field referrals from these groups are at times amazed—and appalled—at what a poor job they sometimes do at managing common skin problems. The near absence of dermatology teaching in medical school explains a lot of this, of course; the standard curriculum imparts not just limited skin knowledge but an implicitly dismissive attitude toward caring for the simple complaints of ordinary people.

There should thus be no surprise at the burgeoning of "physician extenders" (a barbarous term that sounds like "Hamburger Helper"). Physician assistants and nurse practitioners have active professional organizations and a growing membership.

What distinguishes such professionals is that they actually want to do clinical work. They view caring for patients with everyday problems not as a distraction from their main career but as its fulfillment. More and more dermatologists are hiring PA's and NP's to work alongside them.

Professional nature abhors a vacuum. If research provides new treatments, who will administer them? When patients need help, who will take care of them?

PATIENTS

Stacey

Fear concentrates the mind, and nothing causes more fear than the first day of internship. That is one reason I remember Stacey.

The graduating intern was signing out with relief. She briskly assured me that her four patients were all stable: an asthma, a diarrhea, a seizure disorder. Stacey was the last, curled in her crib, a clamped feeding tube protruding from her diaper. Stacey stared into space, twitching spasmodically.

"She has seizures all the time," said the intern. "We told the mother there's no hope she'll recover, and placement would be best. But she didn't listen to us and insisted we put in the feeding tube, because she wants to take her kid home." Letitia, Stacey's mother, stood near the crib with an air of grim determination.

Neurologists had ordered a brain biopsy to see whether a herpes simplex viral infection was the reason a healthy four-year-old had run an unexplained fever of 106 degrees, then lapsed into a two-month coma accompanied by endless jerking of her limbs. The biopsy was negative. Lacking explanations, the doctors were pessimistic and discouraging, but Letitia took Stacey home.

I was assigned to follow Stacey in outpatient clinic. Unlike many other mothers who kept appointments only sporadically, Letitia was as punctual and reliable as she was determined. Each month she brought in her daughter, vacant, rigid, twitching, for my ministrations or advice. She told me what she was feeding Stacey through her feeding tube, and I approved. We spoke of no physical or psychosocial milestones. There were none.

Stacey continued to interest the neurologists. They drew her blood, comparing it to serum they had frozen during her first illness. They found a four-fold rise in the levels of antibodies against vaccinia, the virus used to inoculate against smallpox. Although New York State had abolished routine smallpox vaccination several years before, Stacey's GP inoculated her anyway. This had caused a rare but devastating complication: vaccinia encephalomyelitis. The fact that we had finally established a diagnosis did not present Stacey with any new treatment options or prospects, but did make her case very interesting to those who reviewed and discussed it.

While I was away on vacation eight months later, Stacey once again became suddenly ill. When her temperature rose to 107, Letitia rushed her to the emergency room. Stacey was admitted to the hospital, where she improved and was sent home. No explanation was found for her fever.

After that, Letitia began to notice changes in Stacey. They were subtle, but she was sure she saw them.

Letitia called me soon after, a note of triumph in her voice. She had to bring Stacey in to the clinic. Something was happening. I would see.

The next day Letitia wheeled Stacey toward me through the crowded clinic, locking the wheelchair in front of my curtained cubicle. "Stacey," she commanded, "get up and walk!" And Stacey got up and walked.

At first Stacey was awkward and mute, but then improvement accelerated. Her limbs straightened, her facial features softened. She began to speak. Eleven months after Stacey had lapsed into coma, sophisticated neuropsychological tests could hardly distinguish her from normal. She started school.

The neurologists were amazed. They said that Stacey had set a record for complete recovery after a prolonged coma not induced by trauma. The cause of her illness and its course were both remarkable, they said. We wrote up her case for publication. Letitia moved away, and we lost touch.

I haven't forgotten Stacey, though. Beyond her instructional value as a case of vaccinia brain damage, Stacey taught me about the limits of prediction and the power of hope, two useful lessons for that first, fearful day of internship.

What if Letitia had followed the advice of the experts and had her daughter institutionalized? Would Stacey have improved in the way she finally did, or would neglect have taken its toll and prevented recovery? Did the medical professionals who counseled hopelessness change their approach for later patients, or did they never find out what happened? Even if they did find out, was Stacey's case too unique from which to generalize?

Physicians diagnose, treat, and, more broadly, predict what will happen. As we learn, experience builds confidence. From my very first day, Stacey taught me its limits.

The Invisible Exit Sign

On the wooden door, which leads from my examining room corridor out to the waiting room, a big red sign at eye level reads: "EXIT." This sign is invisible. Time and again patients trying to leave walk up to the door, stare at the sign, then turn left until somebody rescues them and shows them out.

The trouble actually starts sooner. When patients exit the exam room itself, another red sign directly opposite, also at eye level, reads "EXIT," with an arrow pointing to the right. This too is invisible. More than half of patients turn left and soon bump into a blank wall, on which I have placed a sign: "THE WAY OUT IS BEHIND YOU." They ponder this sign—and the blank wall it hangs from. After a short pause for processing, they get the message and turn around.

Since few patients are blind or illiterate, why are my signs invisible? The writing on the signs is plain enough, but they are hanging in an unfamiliar context. When you don't know where you are, you can hardly see anything. To process data, our senses need the help of background cues.

How much such cues matter becomes obvious on trips abroad. When people speak to us in a strange language, we often can't pick up even words we know. Mumbling happens everywhere, but back home we can understand a lot of it because we get the rest of the sentence, know what facial expressions and gestures mean, and so forth.

Patients in our offices are travelers in a strange land. We are so at home that it takes effort to realize how lost they can get in matters of procedure and etiquette, not to mention medical advice. Perhaps we and our staff should think of ourselves as folks who greet tourists at a visitors bureau in a country where people talk funny, act weird, and drive on the wrong side of the road. For instance:

- Check-in: Anyone not experienced in HMO-land can be pardoned for assuming that if you call your primary physician who promises to send a referral, then you've done your job. We know better, of course, but it's fair to be gentle with patients whose referrals haven't come in yet.

- Taking a seat: In my exam rooms, besides the table I have a stool and a chair. I sometimes enter to see a patient sitting in the chair leap to her feet and stammer, "Sorry—I'm in your chair!" It helps if the staff who bring patients into the room tell them where to sit and show them where to hang clothes. (Door hooks are also invisible.)

- Putting on a gown: That you should leave a gown open in back is not self-evident, especially if what worries you is on your front. Proper gowning takes both instruction and demonstration. (Even that may not be enough. At my most recent colonoscopy, they told me to put on *two* johnnies, an upper and a lower—and showed me too—but I still got them wrong. Both of them.)

- <u>Lying down</u>: As everyone knows, if you tell a patient to lie on his back, he will lie on his stomach. If you ask her to lie on her left side, she will turn right.

- <u>Knowing what we do for a living</u>: Just because we know what diagnoses we handle and which procedures we perform, doesn't mean patients do. They ask things like, "Do you take care of warts?" Even more often they apologize because their rash got better or their bleeding spot fell off before they came, assuming that anything less than cancer or complete misery is a waste of our time. It doesn't take much effort to assure them otherwise (or to unintentionally embarrass them by acting bored and dismissive).

- <u>Going for samples</u>: Unless I tell them emphatically to stay put and that I will be *right back*, patients who see me leave to get samples or a liquid nitrogen canister are often overcome by fear of abandonment and come running half-clothed into the hall.

- <u>Understanding instructions</u>: When do you put the cream on? Must you wait after washing? Do you leave it on, or wash it off? And so on and so forth. Many of these directives, self-evident to us, are anything but that to our visitors.

- <u>Exiting</u>: We already covered that.

The bottom line is that when you don't know where you are, almost anything, no matter how simple and obvious, can be inscrutable. Or invisible.

Private Narratives

Someone has published a list of the thirty-six plot lines that cover every dramatic situation. These include: <u>Revenge</u>—Avenger, Criminal (#3); <u>Familial Hatred</u>—Two Family Members Who Hate Each Other (#13); and <u>Adultery</u>—Deceived Spouse, Two Adulterers (#25).

On the list of what motivates people to visit doctors, there are also a limited number of what you might call Master Narratives. As applied to dermatology, some examples are:

- <u>The Beginning of the End</u>: My symptom, however minor, means the start of a process that will lead to death.

- <u>Family Ties</u>: My relative who had this problem suffered or came to a bad end, and because I take after him in looks, personality, and skin type, so will I.

- <u>Unclean! Unclean!</u>: This rash means I am contaminated and will have to remove myself from polite society (or at least my grandchildren). If it's on the penis, it means sex is out indefinitely.

Finding which of these applies to a given patient is useful, because it helps explain why she's actually showed up as opposed to why she says she has. A directed question or two plus a brief, open-ended conversation usually reveal which Master Narratives are at play. For instance:

- "My aunt had exactly the same mole, and it turned cancerous and she died of brain cancer."

- "I haven't been to yoga in a year, because you're lying right next to the next person's foot and I can't have someone else stare at my ugly plantar wart."

Master Narratives are easy to spot, since there are just a few of them, and they apply to many people. Most every patient turns out to be worried on some level that he is dying, allergic, contagious, or ugly. It's therefore helpful to address not just specific symptoms but their implications: by saying that psoriasis is hereditary but doesn't manifest itself the same way in every family member; that warts and fungi are not really very contagious; and so forth.

More tricky are what I call Private Narratives. These are a kind of subplot, significant not to most people but to a particular one. These narratives draw attention to concerns you'd never guess unless you spend an extra minute or two (that's really all it takes) to hear people tell their own story. Here are some examples:

1. Robert complains of a merciless itch that affects just his chest. Nothing odd about itch, but why his chest? Well, it turns out that last October Robert almost died of pericarditis, an inflammation of the tissue surrounding the heart. Not everybody with chest itch thinks he has recurrent pericarditis though, just Robert.

2. Phil has a crusty age spot sticking out of his scalp. Everyone worries when a spot changes, but Phil has a specific concern: this spot is right near the scar where they operated on him twenty-five years ago when he fell off his bike and developed a blood clot on his brain. You'd never guess that unless he told you.

3. Sally's worry about the warts on her left shin seems to go beyond concern that she might spread them by shaving. It turns out that Sally's sister Susie had a skin cancer taken off her left shin.

4. Jeff was at a summer barbeque, netting an impressive collection of juicy mosquito bites on his legs. Why is he so anxious about bug bites? Five years earlier he had a rare condition called vasculitis on his legs, which produces red bumps.

5. Mike has a few red blocked pores in his groin. He also has self-described "Irish Catholic guilt," and a ninety-two-year-old father recovering from prostate surgery. He's been caring for Dad and fears he could spread some kind of infection.

6. Henry has extra pigment on his penis. Is he worried about a sexually transmitted disease? Actually, no. He's worried because his grandfather "had polio or something and got mottled all over."

Some Private Narratives are so specific to an individual that only Holmes-like acuity, or luck, reveal what's actually going on.

Consider Chuck, whose palms are rough and thick. "This started when I cut one palm at my job," he says. "I work at a nuclear plant."

I tell Chuck he has psoriasis, adding that the cut may have triggered its onset but hasn't caused its persistence, much less its appearance on the other palm. "Also," I say, "radioactivity has nothing to do with it."

"You mean I won't glow in the dark?" Chuck laughs. Nervously.

Is Chuck really worried that his palms are radioactive? Actually, yes.

Or consider Becky. Various creams aren't helping her red and scaly lips. This is a common and reasonable concern. Her lips look and feel funny, and she keeps licking them, which makes them worse. People comment, which is embarrassing, especially since lip problems have sexual overtones. But Becky's worries are different.

"I work in a brewery," she says. "If this is some kind of yeast infection, maybe it has to do with beer and I'll have to give up my job."

No one would guess Becky's central fear unless she told them. She'll be happy to ignore her lips—and stop aggravating their redness by nervously licking them—once she knows that every uptick of symptoms doesn't mean unemployment and retraining as an airport baggage scanner.

Personal angles like these come up all the time. Given a minute or two, patients bring them up themselves. Like Phil, who has a thick scar on his chest. He's a middle-aged guy who doesn't seem likely to take his shirt off much. What bothers him about it? Appearance? Fear of cancer?

"I'm a courier for a clinical lab," he says, "so I'm in and out of the car all the time. And every time I fasten my seat belt it rubs this and it hurts."

So that's it—fear of trauma (frequent rubbing could cause cancer, and so forth), but of a very specific and unavoidable sort, given what he does for a living. Easy to address, once you know what the worry is.

But the prize in my collection goes to Harold, who presents with a large cyst on his back. A common enough complaint—why is it there, is it a tumor, etc. But Harold has something specific in mind.

"The bump hurts when I take part in medieval recreations," he says.

"You mean like the Society for Creative Anachronism?" I ask.

"Exactly," says Harold.

For the uninitiated, that society is devoted to recreating the Middle Ages in authentic detail. They put a lot of effort into getting everything just right. This means that the cyst bothers Harold *because it rubs against his armor.*

So he has two choices: to remove the cyst or to wear flexible armor.

Which wouldn't be authentic. So he really has only one choice.

Everyone has a story. They are often well worth the time it takes to listen.

The Exploding Squid
and Other Tales

There was a comic when I was a kid called "The Strange World of Mr. Mum." Each strip featured an impassive gent in a small fedora, who looked on, mum, at the odd things that always seemed to be going on as he passed by, like two masked crooks robbing each other at the same time.

Now and then things happen in my office that make me feel like Mr. Mum. I share them here without comment.

*   *   *   *   *

Tim, a 30-ish architect with sandy hair, had tiny broken blood vessels around his eyes. I asked whether he'd been coughing very hard, or straining at stool. Negative.

I mentally ran through other possibilities. Let's see, too old to be a baby born with the umbilical cord wrapped around his neck...Tim broke into my reverie.

"Doctor, could walking on my hands across the office have anything to do with this?"

"Well…yes, Tim. Would I be out of line to ask *why* you walk across your office on your hands?"

"Oh, I just do it sometimes."

*　　*　　*　　*　　*

Lynn flashed me a conspiratorial look. "Could your student leave the room?"

"Of course." I shooed the student out—they expect that sometimes—wondering what private matter Lynn had to discuss.

"I'm thinking of getting plastic surgery," she said. "Tell me, who did your face?"

"What?!"

"No, really, just between us, I won't tell anybody. Who did your face?"

I managed to regain enough composure to say that I guessed I was flattered, but nobody did my face. She looked skeptical.

I didn't share this exchange with my student, who wouldn't have believed it anyway.

*　　*　　*　　*　　*

At a local medical conference, the guest speaker was giving us a heads-up on ICD-10, the new and improved list of all the diagnosis codes in the medical universe. "It's going to be a lot more detailed than ICD-9," she explained, adding that ICD-10 is slated to become mandatory in October 2013. I heard some murmurs that October

2013 might be a good date to retire.

The speaker flashed several examples of new ICD-10 codes on the screen. "For instance," she said, "this is the code for a benign lesion of the left eyelid. And this [next slide] is the code for a benign lesion of the right eyelid."

A doctor raised his hand. "What difference does it make which lid it's on?" he asked.

Some people just don't get it.

*   *   *   *   *

My heart sank when I entered the exam room and saw the young woman with grotesquely enlarged, hollowed-out earlobes that literally hung to her shoulders. What could she possibly want me to do with them?

Sue was quite pleasant. "See, this is how I make them bigger," she said. "I make a cut at the top, and then put in a larger and larger coin to make the hole bigger until the skin heals around it. Now the earlobes are as big as I want them." Glad to hear that.

"But here's my problem." Sue pointed to a slight protrusion of tissue at the cavity's upper pole, at twelve o'clock. In other words, her problem was not the huge hole—the hole is what she wanted— but the bump at the top that stuck into the cavity and marred its perfection.

"In that case," I said, "I can help you. I'll inject some cortisone into the bump and flatten it."

"Fantastic!" she exclaimed. I gave her the shot, and asked what her career plans were.

"Social work," she explained.

* * * * *

Bob, in for a skin check, had a healing scab on his forehead. "Looks like you ran into a pipe and didn't duck fast enough," I suggested.

"Not exactly," said Bob. "I was making squid and shrimp pasta in the microwave. When all the pieces got nice and plump, I decided to test whether they were done, so I stuck a fork into one of the squid, and it exploded. Guess I was lucky it didn't get my eye."

I guessed he was. Microwave-induced exploding cats are said to be urban legends, but now we know that exploding squid have been sighted in real life. Doctors, take note! Do not forget to ask your patients whether they have been attacked by an exploding squid, as well as whether they walk on their hands across their offices (or stand on their heads doing yoga).

I'll take my fedora off, for now.

Self-Absorption

Irma had a few spots on her face. I told her I could freeze them off.

"This may not be a good time," she said. "I'm going to a professional convention this weekend, and I don't want to be self-conscious."

"That's all right," I said. "Maybe when you have vacation coming up."

"No, any other week will be fine."

"But won't your patients notice?"

"Probably not," she said. "They're too self-absorbed."

Irma is a psychologist.

Her observation is striking, because it contrasts so strongly with what most people say about the reactions they get when there is something noticeable on their faces. Irma may think her patients will be indifferent, but teachers and relatives of small children expect the opposite. Children don't know much about tact.

"WHAT IS THAT UGLY THING ON YOUR CHIN, MRS. DONNELLY?" the kids yell. Grandparents tell similar stories about their little darlings. ("Nana, why do you have those bumps on your neck? I hate them!") Enduring enough of those comments is often what drives people to ask for removing growths that haven't bothered them for decades.

All of us have a very strong urge to point out blemishes, especially on the face—a red mark, a piece of food hanging off our dining partner's lower lip. Not commenting takes ferocious self-control. Not noticing takes an awful lot of self-absorption.

But some people rise to the self-absorptive occasion in other ways too. For instance, one of my colleagues collaborates with a plastic surgeon based in his office two days a week. The surgeon developed acute abdominal pain one night and was rushed to a local emergency room. When a CT scan showed appendicitis, he was taken to the OR first thing in the morning. My friend's secretary started calling the surgeon's patients to let them know that their consultations or surgeries would need to be postponed.

Most people reacted with appropriate concern. ("Oh, I'm so sorry to hear that! How is he doing?" and so on.) But not everyone.

"I'm sorry to tell you that Dr. Jenkins won't be able to see you today. He's having emergency surgery himself."

"Oh. I see. That's *very* disappointing."

"Of course. But we'll let you know as soon as we find out when he's coming back to work."

"This is *very* disappointing."

Alas, so it is.

Or another: a man had flown up from Florida for another opinion about biopsy-proven skin cancer. The second opinion was the same as the first—that the cancer be removed. An expedited consultation was arranged with the surgeon so the Floridian could go right back to the sun. When appendicitis struck the surgeon, the patient was apprised of the situation.

"But when will Dr. Jenkins be able to operate?" he wanted to know.

"He's in surgery himself right now," he was told. "We hope he recovers fast, but at this point we really can't tell you."

"But I have to make plans," he said. "When will he be able to take care of my problem?"

What the secretary thought of saying—but didn't—was, "Tell you what. We'll camp out in the recovery room with an iPhone next to Dr. Jenkins's lips. The second his anesthesia wears off, we're sure his very first words—after he asks about his mistress—will be to tell us when he can operate on you."

Talk about self-absorption.

Of course, we meet self-absorbed people in all walks of life. And all of us—even doctors!—are entitled to think about our own pressures and problems, though sharing them with patients is generally not a good move. ("You think *you've* got a rash? Have a look at *mine*!") It's okay to be annoyed when your doctor, lawyer, or accountant can't see you as scheduled, but most people older than a certain age can see the larger context and stifle the urge to express their annoyance.

I saw Irma again after her convention and froze her offending spots. "I guess from what you told me," I said, "your self-absorbed patients won't even notice."

"I'm not sure my colleagues at the convention would have noticed either," she said, with a wry smile. "They're psychologists."

Look, *she* said it, I didn't.

Lost to Follow-Up

Rosalie hadn't been by in three years. Her chief concern was a growth on her forearm. Then she pointed to a cholesterol deposit above her right eye. "I thought it might have been from crying," she said. "My daughter died fourteen months ago. She was twenty-six."

I expressed sympathy, and asked if her daughter had been ill. "It's a long story," she said, "but the short of it is that she had a boyfriend who was not a good person. He stored a gun in her closet, and she didn't even know it was there. One night she came home after going out drinking with her girlfriends, other nurses from the hospital. She tripped in the closet, and the gun went off.

"She used to be your patient," Rosalie said. "Maybe you remember, she got those crazy warts when she was in middle school." I checked my records. Her daughter's last visit was fifteen years ago, when she was thirteen.

In our offices, as elsewhere in our lives, people pass across our line of vision and disappear. We may find out what becomes of them, medically or otherwise, but more often we don't. Sometimes a chance encounter brings their image back into focus, but for the most part once out of sight they stay out of mind.

This is true not just of patients like Rosalie's daughter who come a time or two for a minor complaint, but also for those we get to know over a sustained period. All at once you realize that you haven't seen them lately, and perhaps never will again.

Terry is so familiar that I was surprised to see she hadn't come for over a year. Now past eighty, she looked a bit frailer than the last time I saw her but still reasonably hale. I recalled that Tim, her husband and inseparable companion, had no longer come along to her last couple of visits. Tim wasn't up to it, she'd explained. His mind was getting a little fuzzy. He sent his regards.

This time I asked Terry about him with some hesitation. Dementia, after all, may advance in fits and starts, but goes in just one direction. "He's doing fairly well," she said. "Lately when Tim sees women on the TV, he thinks they can see him, so he won't undress in the bedroom because he's embarrassed. I tell him, 'Timmy, why aren't you worried that the men in the TV can see me?' But he still won't get into his pajamas until I turn off the TV.

"During the day he's pretty content," she went on. "He just sits there by his radio, all day long. He loves to listen to it and look out the window. He can sit there for hours. Then I remind him that it's time to eat, and afterwards he goes back to his radio, and listens."

Terry's report jogged my memory of the way Tim looked when I saw him last, an affable gent, with a wiry build and thinning brown hair. He always had a smile on his face, ready to help me reassure his wife, the worrier of the pair. At the end of each visit I would wish them good health and say I looked forward to seeing them next year.

Now that I won't be seeing him anymore, I'll have to picture Tim in Terry's description, listening to his murmuring radio and gazing out the window as he subsides into his own deepening twilight.

Of course it's not only patients who pass by and are lost to follow-up. People come to the office and tell me they had a physical or biopsy as recently as two or three years ago, but cannot for the life of them remember which doctor they saw. It's even not unusual for someone to come back to me after an absence of a decade or two and express disbelief that they'd ever been here, since neither the office nor its proprietor rang a bell.

When I was starting out in practice, an older colleague told me that once he announced his retirement, his mailbox filled and his phone rang off the hook with messages from anguished patients declaring that they simply would not be able to get along without him. "They did manage, though," he said. "In most cases it took only a couple of weeks."

Obsession

I was about to desiccate some small keratoses on Edwin's face.

"Will this scar, Doctor? Will it leave a hole?"

"No, it won't scar or leave a hole."

"Will it leave a scar or a hole?"

"No. No scar or hole."

"Will it leave a scar or a hole?"

"No scar. No hole."

Obsessives present a challenge. It's hard to answer the same question over and over without being tempted to slug the questioner. This impulse should be resisted.

Because of the kind of work we do, dermatologists encounter obsessive behavior rather often, whether or not it rises to the level of clinical obsessive-compulsive disorder (OCD). Its roots can be the patient's anxiety, social role, or personal style.

Anxiety is a great promoter of obsession.

"This spot is changing. Is it cancer?"

"No, it isn't cancer."

"It's not cancer?"

"It's not cancer."

"Are you sure it's not cancer?"

By this point we may be wondering how sure we are, but we can't very well say, "Well, okay, maybe it is cancer," without losing a certain credibility.

Then there is social role, specifically the maternal one. Mothers feel required to make sure no stone is left unturned, for fear that later, one of the stones will turn out to have something under it. This leads to familiar family mini-dramas.

"Samantha, please take off your shoe and show the doctor your warts. Do you have some on the other foot, Samantha?"

"No, Ma, just on this one."

"Why not take off your other shoe, just to check."

"There aren't any on the other foot. I looked."

"We're at the doctor's. Let's take a look, to be sure."

"Ma!"

Someday Samantha will get her chance to pay this forward.

Then there is personal style. It's beyond my competence to decide which of such patients deserves the diagnostic label of OCD, just as I am unsure how many people who admit to washing their hands ten or fifteen times a day are more than just fastidious. In any case, obsessive style can show itself in making lists, whether of complaints or spots.

Our hearts sink, of course, at the sight of a meticulous list of concerns. "I wrote down my questions, Doctor, so I won't forget any."

Questions on lists are best addressed individually and in order. Any deviation means having to start over. ("Wait, did we do this one yet?") This is especially true when the list contains specific spots to look at. Each listed spot must be noted and addressed individually. Global evaluations will not do.

"It's on my back somewhere."

"Let's see. I'm looking at your whole back, and everything looks fine."

"But wait, it's here somewhere…"

If the patient is sufficiently anxious or obsessional, I resort to what I call "the OCD three-step." I touch the spot, pause, and say:

"I'm looking at it…I can see it…and it's okay."

Only then may I move on to the next spot. Any change in sequence or cadence means having to start over. ("Wait, did you see it?")

Once they finger a spot, patients tend to fondle it lovingly—and at length—making it necessary to gently suggest that they move their opaque digit out of the way.

Sometimes, of course, people can't find what worries them, especially when it is on a hard-to-detect area like the scalp. If there is something more maddening than watching someone palpate himself with increasingly desperate and furious futility, I don't know what it is. When this happens, I politely excuse myself and leave the room, explaining that identifying the spot will be easier when I'm not standing there making everyone nervous. Then I return a couple of minutes later to find the beaming patient with his index finger affixed to his noggin. "I found it!" he exclaims.

Ah, blessed relief.

Compared with our colleagues who may have to address complex medical issues, dermatologists have a pretty easy time of it overall. Dealing with obsessive behavior can be a challenge, but one that's generally manageable as long as we don't get two or three such patients in a row. That circumstance calls for some form of tension relief, perhaps a glass of something or other after hours. That's what I think, anyhow.

So what do you think?

So what do you think?

So what do you think?

Lost in Translation

The first language of many of my patients is not English. Some of those who speak Spanish or Russian come with a family member or friend to translate. This sometimes leads to odd situations.

Yesterday, for instance, Olga brought in her elderly mother and father. I examined them and offered my opinion. "Let me tell them what you think," Olga said, and began to address her parents. They listened with rapt attention until I interrupted her and said, "Excuse me, Olga, but you're speaking English." She looked confused, then smiled, gave her forehead a little slap, and talked to them in Russian.

I've managed to pick up some Russian myself. I don't have much of a vocabulary, just a few words and phrases, and not necessarily those you'd learn with Berlitz but the ones a dermatologist might find helpful, like *da svidaniye* (see you later), *spasibo* (thank you), *borodavka* (wart), *grybok* (fungus), *ni rak* (it isn't cancer), and *kho key* (okay!).

Once I was speaking with an elderly Russian man who had toenail fungus. Eager to communicate and show what I knew, I said,

"Mr. Serebrennikov, on your toenails you have *grybok*." His face brightened. "That's amazing!" he said. "We have the same word in Russian!"

Da svidaniye!

Denial

Stella seems like a sensible woman. Because she's had two skin cancers removed, she comes regularly for me to check her sun-damaged skin.

About four years ago I prevailed on Stella to let me examine her in full, something she had insisted wasn't necessary. I was almost done when I looked under her bra and noticed something. Further inspection showed both her breasts completely covered with red, eroded skin. Taken aback, I asked her how long this had been there.

"Oh, about a month," she said, indifferently.

Not terribly likely. Biopsy showed Paget's disease, an uncommon form of breast cancer. She had this treated with surgery and radiation. Stella continues to see me once a year, and still gives the impression of being level-headed and sensible.

But I have to ask myself: all that time (months? years?), whenever she undressed or showered and saw her ugly and disfigured breasts, what was she thinking? That they were supposed to look that way? That they would heal by themselves? That what was staring her in the face really wasn't there?

I ask myself the same about Robert, an amiable if absent-minded philosophy professor with a bushy red beard. Underneath the hair on his left cheek he had a gaping, oozing hole. Who knows how long that had been there. Although his beard made this chasm—which turned out to be a huge basal cell skin cancer—invisible to onlookers, even professors wash their faces now and then. What was Robert thinking when he touched or saw this repulsive defect, which measured several centimeters in diameter by the time he showed up in my office? That oozing holes belong on the face?

Like Stella, Robert readily agreed to take care of his cancer. He follows up regularly, showing no sign of being delusional, or even much odder than the average philosophy professor.

Denial is indeed a powerful thing. It helps people ignore what is right before their eyes.

I can think back over the years to spectacular instances like those of Stella and Robert, patients who let visible cancers grow and fester for decades. Twenty years ago a patient phoned. "My wife is coming to see you," he said, "and I want you to know in advance that we're aware we have a problem, and we're working on it." I asked him what he was talking about. "We've been married twelve years," he said, "and she's never taken off her shirt."

His wife turned out to be a globetrotting business executive in her mid-thirties's. She showed me a basal cell cancer that extended from her mid-chest to her left shoulder. This ended up needing both surgery and radiation.

But there have also been many less dramatic examples of people who just couldn't be bothered to take care of things they knew they had to treat, or follow up on what they agreed they ought to. Some claimed they were too busy, others were clearly afraid of bad news. So they looked at themselves with eyes wide shut.

Doctors simply can't assume our patients will act in their own best interests, that they will get a skin cancer removed because we told them they have one, or that they will come back regularly because they're at high risk. Beyond making a recommendation, we need to check whether they followed it and badger them if they haven't.

I sometimes shrug when experts, from economists to ethicists, describe people as rational actors who make sound decisions to advance their interests as long as they have the proper data with which to do so. I wonder which people they have in mind. They obviously can't mean Stella and Robert, and a lot of other people I meet every day.

Denial is so easy, after all. In many aspects of life it's simple to manage not to notice that you're behaving in ways that make health, finances, or relationships worse instead of better. Much simpler, surely, than not seeing skin rotting away before your eyes.

Show Me Your Paw

The man had an innocuous, American-sounding name. Let's call him Al Morse. Al lives in New Hampshire. It's midwinter, and Al says he's taking his wife dog-sledding.

"Ever done the Iditarod?" I ask.

"Been to Alaska lots of times," he says. Then he adds, "Thing is, my dogs only understand Ukrainian or Russian. You tell 'em 'Sit!' and they don't know what you're talking about. But say, '*Sydity!*' and they sit right down.

"I learned how to talk to these dogs from my folks," says Al. "My people are from Dnepropetrovsk." He then launches into a series of (to me) flawlessly-accented Ukrainian sled-dog commands, my favorite (though not in Ukrainian) being, "Show me your paw."

I doubt I'll ever ask a Slavic sled-dog to show me its paw, but knowing that Al does may give me insight if my team ever looks perplexed. Picking up tips like this helps me reflect on what a wonderful profession medicine can be. You meet people you'd never otherwise run into, and find out about things they do that you never imagined existed and couldn't make up.

Take Mr. Blanchard, a middle-aged gent not currently employed who lives in Revere, just north of Boston. Mr. Blanchard, who has the kind of rolling baritone favored by earlier generations of radio announcers, has a deep love of two Old Testament books: Ecclesiastes and Job. That this pair is among the most depressing ever written does not dampen his enthusiasm for them. Mr. Blanchard says he has committed to memory every available English translation of each. He will cite quotations at the drop of a hat, or even if a hat doesn't drop.

Every morning at dawn Mr. Blanchard strides along Revere Beach and declaims Ecclesiastes and Job to the waves. He says this does great things for his lungs and gets his day started out right, though what you would feel like doing with your day after digesting the wisdom of Job and Ecclesiastes is not clear. Perhaps you'd have a donut. (Of making donuts there is no end.)

"It's inspiring," says Mr. Blanchard, with gusto, "to look out over the waves and say, as Job did, 'All the rivers flow into the sea, yet the sea is not full.'"

I gently observe that this is Ecclesiastes. If you're going to limit your canon to two books, you might as well keep them straight.

I could not invent Mr. Blanchard. Yet I have met him.

And then just the other day Kevin comes in with his mother. A wrestler, Kevin has contracted a loathsome scalp infection now oozing south-southeast onto his forehead. Knowing how mothers often feel about their sons engaging in contact sports, I gibe, "How about taking up chess, Kevin?"

"I do chess boxing," he says, not missing a beat.

"What?"

"Chess boxing," he repeats. "It's really popular. First you make some chess moves, then you box, and you go back and forth. You win either by a checkmate or a knockout."

"What on earth are you talking about?" I respond. I figure this kid for the slickest leg-puller I ever met. But he seems quite sincere.

Later, I Google "chess boxing," and wouldn't you know that it's right there on Wikipedia (where else?). The article begins:

> **Chess boxing** is a hybrid sport, which combines boxing with chess in alternating rounds. The sport began when Dutch artist Iepe Rubingh, inspired by fictional depictions by French comic book artist and filmmaker Enki Bilal, organized actual bouts. Chess boxing is now growing in popularity. Participants must be both skilled boxers and chess players, as a match may be won either way.

It includes a photo of a 2008 Berlin match, with two boxers in a distant ring and a chess set close-up in the foreground.

Are my colleagues going to tell me they didn't know about chess boxing? What do they do—spend all their time reading medical journals? They should get out more. Or learn from their patients, who do.

Ecclesiastes wrote that there is nothing new under the sun. But Ecclesiastes didn't know about chess boxing, did he?

I must call Mr. Blanchard as soon as he gets back from his walk. If he has a dog, I wonder what languages it responds to.

Skating Along the Surface

One day in late August I was explaining to Maria how to apply hydroquinone to the extra pigmentation on her upper lip.

"It will work better after Labor Day," I said, "when the sun isn't so strong. Please apply it morning and night, and be sure to use sunscreen whenever you go outdoors. I'll see you back in two months."

"I may be in the sun then," she said. "I probably will be taking my son to Disney. He has leukemia, and the doctors say they can't do anything more for him."

I was speechless. Here I was, discoursing on lip pigment to a woman planning Christmas in October for her little son on the brink of death.

"Edgar got sick when he was ten months old," Maria went on. "The medicines helped for a while. Now he's seven. But they're not working anymore. So we're going to take him to Disney."

Like everyone, all our patients have stories. Some have several: banal, amusing, frustrating, tragic. At times we can infer them from their skin complaints, or from conversational byplay during visits. Mostly, however, we treat the superficialities, with barely any idea of what goes on underneath. It could hardly be otherwise; what's down there is not our business. And how much can you learn in a few minutes assigned to the integument?

Then someone like Maria comes along, to remind us of how limited our role actually is, how little we understand the people we take care of, how trifling, in the larger scheme of things, are the therapies we have at our disposal.

Once I had two such reminders on the same day. Laurel brought in Emma, her chunky five-year-old. That Emma had eczema was evident from her scaly arms even before she reached the exam table. Laurel herself shuffled in, looking unkempt and disheveled. She had dirty, two-inch nails. Her skin was sallow, her voice grating. A smoker who didn't take care of herself, no doubt. "Emma, get up on the table and sit still!" she rasped.

"Emma has eczema," I told her. "I'll give you some cream for it."

"Thanks, Doc," she said. "I'm trying to get things straightened out for her as much as I can. I have Lou Gehrig's disease, or at least that's what the doctors think. They've been running tests for six months. That's why I talk like this.

"I don't know how much longer I'm going to be able to take care of her. But there isn't anybody else. I have no family. There's just me." She forced herself clumsily to her feet.

"It's a hard life," she said, lurching over to help Emma down. I handed her the prescription for a topical steroid. That is all I had to offer.

A few hours later a waif came in, accompanied by an attendant from an agency. The chart said Ellen was twelve, though she looked no more than eight. Even a cursory glance made it plain that Ellen was gouging herself. Fresh wounds marred her arms, alongside healed scars. Common enough in adults; not so much in a child.

"I scratch myself," she said. "My psychiatrist is helping me with that."

"Does your skin itch?" I asked.

"Sometimes," she said. "But sometimes I just get nervous. It depends on my foster parents. When I'm with a new family it takes me a while to feel at home. I worry that maybe they won't like me, and I'll have to move again.

"But now I'm in a good home!" She spoke with urgency, as though trying to convince herself. "Everyone's really very nice. So I'm hoping I can stay with them for a while. And when I feel good, I don't pick at my skin so much."

Once again I prescribed something, which is what I was expected to do. An application as an alternative to self-mutilation. Her psychiatrist could work on her self-esteem, even as her circumstances dismantled what was left of it.

Cases like these are, of course, exceptional. For the most part ours is a cheerful specialty. Patients are happy or can be made so. Such stresses as we get wind of—a lost job, parent-teenager tensions— are mild and conventional, or at least they seem that way to us.

As outsiders, we have a conveniently limited role. We offer our superficial ministrations, skating blithely along the surface.

Ménage

Call me old-fashioned, but I'm just not comfortable talking with young women about their sexual practices. Particularly when their mothers are in the room. Sometimes, of course, there is no choice. Before prescribing a drug like Isotretinoin that causes severe birth defects if taken while pregnant, one simply has to know whether a woman is sexually active, and if so, what kind of contraception she practices.

It's interesting, though, and a sign of how times have changed, that any discomfort involved in such discussions seems limited to me. Neither daughters nor their mothers seem troubled at all, either by questions about sex or by the answers they prompt.

There was Nataliya, for instance, a college student home for intersession. Next to the examining table, her mother sat knitting.

At Nataliya's request, I examined a new bump on her privates. It was a wart. Of course I needed to know whether any partners had warts too, or if her partners were women, whether they had been examined internally to find out.

Old-fashioned though I am, I do recognize the need to speak in gender-neutral terms. "Does your partner have warts?" I asked.

"I don't think so," she said.

That didn't tell me what I needed to know, so I tried again, this time more directly. "Is your partner a man?" I asked.

No answer.

"Is your partner a woman?"

Still no answer.

"Nataliya, it's generally one or the other," I said.

There was a long pause. Finally, Nataliya spoke. "Both," she said.

Of course! Why hadn't I thought of that?

"It's a married couple," she continued. "I feel terrible to have to tell them. I'm very close to both of them."

I guess so, I thought. But I managed not to express overt surprise. You learn something new every day.

What struck me was not so much my own naïveté, but the fact that during this interchange Nataliya's mother did not react at all. Her continued calm seemed consistent with hearing her daughter comment on the weather.

Most college girls (and boys) don't come to the doctor with their parents to talk about genital issues. You might have thought that Nataliya's mom's showing up implied unfashionable, old world over-protectiveness. But then, you might have been wrong to think so.

Pondering Nataliya brought to mind an incident that happened almost thirty years ago. On my way out of town with my wife and young children, I stopped at the hospital for a consultation. The patient was seventeen, accompanied at the bedside by her mother. Examining the teen, I saw what I had only seen in textbooks and have never encountered again: gonorrhea in the bloodstream, showing itself on the skin of the ankle.

"I don't know how to tell you this," I stammered. "But I think we need to order a culture for gonorrhea."

"Tell me, Doc," said the mother. "My daughter and I had sex with the same man. Did I give this to her?"

I said no and left as fast as I could to write my chart note and rejoin my family. Then too the only embarrassed person in the room had been me.

But as I said, I am old-fashioned.

You Missed a Spot!

I thought I'd seen everything, until Jack took off his shirt. On his chest, back, and arms were a dozen round stickers, each the canary color of smiley faces. What now? Day-Glo nicotine patches?

Jack explained. "The last time you took off my age spots," he said, "you missed a few. So I marked them." Sure enough, next to each sticker a brown excrescence glared like a crusty reproach. No way I'd miss those babies this time.

Now I was back on familiar ground. Over the years I've seen patients mark spots that concern them with:

- ink dots next to spots

- ink circles around spots

- mascara circles around spots

- crude but elaborate anatomical drawings, studded with dots. (I keep some in my files—they could be worth something some day.)

- narrative descriptions written in the style of treasure

maps. ("Go three inches above the left third knuckle, turn right...")

This is not satire. This is my life.

Many patients have obsessional tendencies which make them show up with lists—of questions, of spots—which they absolutely must get through, into, and in order before life can go on. One or two such patients can be amusing, annoying, challenging, or maddening. Three in a row, and I need a stiff scotch.

When it comes to concerns like these about spots, the distinction between "medical" and "cosmetic" is irrelevant. It matters not whether the offending spots are skin tags, warts, or solar keratoses (precancerous). People point to and lovingly massage each one in turn, because a spot mars their surface and offends them the same way that a piece of tomato hanging off your dining partner's lip does, or a run in your hose, or a scratch on the hood of your shiny new car. The lip, stocking, and car work just fine, but there's a spot on them and you've got to get it off!

Over the years I've developed strategies to deal with patients with lists of spots or questions.

1. *Get hold of that list!* Gently extract the slip of paper, and tick off the items one by one. This helps spare your anxious patient the chore of rereading over and over the ones you already covered, fearful that maybe you missed one. This has gotten harder, as more people arrive with lists on their cellphones.

2. *Wait till the list is done.* This may be hard, especially if the list is memorized and you don't know how long it's going to be. You

can tell a lot by body language, however. As you go from point to point, or spot to spot, patients will stay tense and hunched over, with a look of fear and anxiety lest something get skipped. Trying to wrap things up before they're done will make them angry and resentful. Thus distracted, they may forget one, then call or return with a reproachful, "You missed a spot!" Actually, many patients soften their critique by saying, "I think *we* missed a spot." We're in this together!

3. *Be specific.* Don't just look at the back and say, "Everything here looks all right." Instead, point at each spot in particular and comment on it. You must specify that you saw exactly what was worrying the patient (or spouse) and announce that it doesn't worry you. For especially obsessive people, I advise using this three-part formula: "I am looking at this spot. I can see it. And it's okay." Only when you say all three—in order!—will he relax.

4. *Have patients mark their spots at home.* Even laid-back people can't find what they're looking for and become anxious and agitated when an impatient, white-coated figure is standing over them with a spray can of liquid nitrogen or an electric needle. That's a guarantee that you'll miss a spot. (Okay, both of you will miss the spot.) If patients want you to scour their integument on a search-and-destroy mission, ask them to spend a few minutes the night before in the comfort of their own bedroom marking off what they want done or looked at. That way they can't blame you for sloppiness. Tell them they can use ink, marker, or mascara. Or yellow stickers.

Incoherence

One after the other, both women came in for skin checks. Oh, but there was so much more. There always is.

I asked Doris about her overall medical condition.

"I'm feeling much better," she said. "I had what I can only call a brain fog. I couldn't concentrate, and I had no interest in doing any of the things I used to enjoy. I don't know how I could have gotten it, but they diagnosed chronic Lyme disease. My doctor was at a loss. As you know, the AMA doesn't know what to do with that diagnosis." (She said this with a smile.) "I went to a chiropractor north of Boston. Then I found a practitioner in Vermont, and when she retired she sent me to someone else. Finally I found an MD Naturopath in Portland, Maine. He offered me two options. The first one, long-term intravenous antibiotics, didn't sound very good, so I chose the second, a diet meant to boost my immune system. And it worked! I feel so much better. He wants me to avoid gluten, and I do, but I really love bread and pasta. So I still eat them sometimes, but not as much.

"Maybe it's all in my head," she mused. "Maybe I just want to think that boosting my immune system makes me feel better, but whatever the reason, the fog is gone and I feel like myself again." Her skin exam was normal.

The next patient was Irene, who listed her medications as Etanercept and Methotrexate, two heavy-duty medications used for severe psoriasis and for arthritis, and other debilitating conditions as well. Seeing no psoriasis or much debilitation for that matter, I asked what those medicines were for.

"Arthritis," she said. "I've been taking them for three years. Before that I was on Adalimumab."

"And that didn't help?"

"It worked, I guess, but I thought maybe something else would work better. I'm not sure if the new treatment does, but I stay on it anyway. My legs are still very swollen, see?"

They didn't look very swollen to me.

"When I get achy, I also take ibuprofen," she said. "And I go to an acupuncturist and do yoga."

You have to love people. (Actually, if you're a physician it's nice if you do.) People are so wonderfully insistent on interpreting for themselves what is wrong with them and how they are doing. And they are so cheerfully incoherent.

Does Doris believe in Western medicine? Well, she's in the office of someone who practices it. Does she believe in chiropractic? Naturopathy? Yes, maybe, sometimes. How about Irene. What is her position on acupuncture? Yoga? Does either patient know the theories behind any of these healing systems? Would pointing out the mutual incompatibility of these theories trouble Irene and Doris? Not for a moment. Whatever works—or seems to.

This is hidden from their many respective practitioners, all of whom are sure their own ministrations are working. They may never even find out that their patient is using other therapies, since patients are reluctant to allude to the competition.

Doris thinks she is on a gluten-free diet, sort of, but of course she does eat some bread and pasta. Practicing clergy will smile in recognition of this kind of behavior. How many of their flock have nibbled at the fruit of the gluten (it tastes good!), only not that often and not so much (nobody's perfect!), without a trace of concern that backsliding implies they've resigned membership in the community of the faithful. Being incoherent means never having to say that non-compliance shows you've quit.

I love incoherence. People who insist on believing just one thing to the exclusion of all others tend to be humorless, self-righteous scolds. Tough to deal with. I stay as far away from them as circumstances allow.

Our own medical world grows increasingly rational and bureaucratized. All is aimed at being neat, tidy, and objective, cataloguing outcomes research and evidence-based therapies, filling centralized data banks with meticulous, often pseudo-precise categories that will include in the next iteration one code for skin tags of the left eyelid and another for the right. There is something to applaud in this trend, which contributes to advancing science and discarding useless traditions.

Oh, but there is more! There has always been so much more than is dreamt of in all this. And, whether or not anyone bothers to admit it, there always will be.

Making Sense of People

Like many who work with the public, I often get the chance to see how little sense people can make. Even so, last week was unusual.

On Tuesday I saw Beulah, who hadn't been here in eight years. "I showed Doctor Prince this spot on my leg," she said. "It's been there a month, and I'm worried about it."

"Just a blocked follicle," I told her. "Put some antibiotic ointment on it, and it will be fine."

Beulah sighed with relief. "I don't need another cancer," she said. "I already have stomach cancer. Doctor Prince told me I couldn't have surgery or other treatment, because I wouldn't make it through. But I'm ninety-eight years old, and I guess we all have to go sometime. I don't have any family left. They're all gone.

"I've lost thirty pounds," she said, still spry enough to hop off the exam table. "None of my clothes fit anymore. But it's awfully good to hear that I don't have to worry about that spot on my leg."

"That is a relief," I agreed.

The next morning I greeted Iris warmly. "How are those

grandchildren?" she asked, as she always does. "Do you have any new pictures?"

"I thought you were moving to Florida, Iris," I said.

"It's been a tough year," she said, "so I had to come back." She went on to tell me how her husband had become jaundiced and succumbed in less than three months to cancer of the bile duct. "It's crazy, Doctor," she said. "Both his brothers have cancer, they had operations years ago, and they're fine. My husband was never sick a day in his life, never even had to take Tylenol for a headache. And now he's gone."

We talked about Iris's own problem, scleroderma, which is all but untreatable and usually fatal but somehow in her case was not progressing at all. Her only skin complaint, easily disposed of, was mild hand eczema.

After some further pleasantries and picture showing, Iris took out a bag of skin care products. "I'm running low on these," she said. "Is there any way I could get some while I'm here?"

Sure she could.

Then on Thursday Sybil came by, a robust woman of seventy-nine who wanted some pigmented lesions checked. As I looked her over, I asked about her family.

"My baby brother has Lewy body dementia," she said. "He's not doing very well. He's in a nursing home now, because his family couldn't take care of him anymore. He still recognizes us a little, or seems to, when we come to visit. It's very painful to watch."

Then Sybil brightened, pointing to the brown spots on the backs of her hands. "Can we laser these off?" she asked. "I really hate them."

Of course we can.

By week's end I was really perplexed. How do people do that, I wondered. How can they go from the profound to the trivial with no acknowledgment, no apology, no "I know this will sound frivolous after what I just told you?" How do they manage such a sudden and seamless register change as if they don't notice the difference, as though an opera singer stopped mid-aria and launched into "Jingle Bells" without so much as a wink.

But they do. I am just about gone, they say, I have outlived everyone around, but what a relief that I don't have skin cancer. My husband just died a painful and senseless death, but I need those creams to help my skin look younger. My little brother is wasting away before my eyes, and how about those pesky age spots?

On reflection, such paradoxes may be more apparent than real. Unless we succumb to deep depression or utter despair, we want to go on living. This means setting aside gloomy thoughts, even if just for a while, and attending to all matters, profound or trivial, that people pay attention to until we give up altogether.

Since no one can make tragedy go away, I guess it's nice to be able to mitigate its impact just a little, around the edges, now and then.

But the end of last week left me shaking my head. I hope never to stop trying, but I doubt that I'll ever really understand people as long as I live.

Cheaper Insurance

Yvette is a striking woman. She wears striking clothes, and her large handbag is boldly accented with what could be gold. Her bronzed, wrinkled skin testifies to five decades of dedicated sun exposure. So do her several squamous cell carcinomas.

I sent her to a plastic surgical colleague for excision of her newest cancer, this one on her chest, explaining that there would have to be a scar but a plastic surgeon would minimize it. The problem was Yvette's low-paying health insurance plan, one that's unpopular among plastic surgeons, to say the least.

"Could you put in a good word for me?" Yvette asked. "Maybe the surgeon could get credentialed on my insurance?" I promised to ask.

Two weeks later Yvette was back, this time to show me a new spot, so that the surgeon could do both if necessary. "By the way," she said, "the surgeon got credentialed on my insurance. Isn't that lovely? Most doctors wouldn't do that nowadays."

I agreed. "I had to go on this new insurance I have," Yvette said. "Blue Cross was just too expensive. I saved over $100 a month by switching."

I told her I'd call with biopsy results. Not long after, I spoke with the surgeon, whom I complimented for agreeing to join Yvette's plan.

"No problem," said the surgeon. "Besides, I like dealing with Yvette. Every time she comes in, she drops a thousand or two on fillers or cosmetic work."

While I Have You

Good morning, Doctor. I haven't seen you in a year, and I have so many questions to discuss. Here, I wrote them down, so I won't forget any. They're all pretty minor, or at least I hope so.

Let's see. This spot here on my left shin? You froze it last year but it didn't go away. There's another one just like it on the other leg. They look the same but I sometimes feel a pain under this one on the left, and the one on the right sometimes itches. Could that mean anything?

And here's another spot near my right elbow. Right now it looks brown, but occasionally it looks red. I put cream on it, which seems to help sometimes but not always. I think it was the cream you gave me last year, but it could be the cream my primary doctor gave me a couple of years ago for a rash. I didn't bring it with me, but it might be at home. It's in a tube. I think it has a green stripe on it, or maybe yellow. If the red spot comes back, should I use the cream again?

Let me look at my list. Oh, yes, look right here, below my right armpit. You can see it if I twist this way—yes, there it is. Now what's really interesting is that my mother and sister have exactly the same mole. Isn't that amazing? Do you think it should be removed? My sister had it removed, but my mother left hers alone. I take after my sister in a lot of ways, but I have my mother's skin. My brother does too, but not my other sister.

And here is something really interesting. You see this area here, on my side? There was a spot there. You can't see it, but it was there two weeks ago, which is why I made the appointment. I was at a party at the house of a friend of a friend. I've been there once or twice, but I'm not that familiar with the layout. I like the hostess, but not her husband that much. Anyhow, I went into the kitchen to get something to drink. They just had the kitchen redone, it looks like it cost them a fortune. Anyway, I bumped into the new island and hit that part of my body. It hurt for a while—I guess that would make sense, since I hit it—but when I looked for the spot the next day, I couldn't find it. Isn't that interesting? So I was wondering whether a spot could just fall off like that and whether hitting it could cause some sort of problem. I know I shouldn't pick at things, but sometimes it's an accident and I can't help it.

Okay, that should be about it. Let me see, did I already ask you about the one in my armpit? Yes, I think I did. So there are really only a couple of more areas I was concerned about. There's this spot on my right ear. Yes, over there. And a dark area on my left ankle...no, not there, right there. Let me turn over the page, I have a few more questions. And I have a funny sensation near my navel, but only sometimes. I know, I can't see anything either, but it bothers me when the weather changes.

I guess that's my whole list. Let's see...wait, did I ask you about the spot on my leg? Yes, I think I did. You're sure the pain isn't related to the spot? Okay, let me turn over the paper again. That may be it...let me just check, as long as I have you. Okay, let me see now. That should be about it. Let me just double-check. Yes, we talked about that, and that. And that. Right, that one. Okay, I guess we're done. I appreciate your taking the time to answer all my questions. Yes, I hope you have a pleasant year too. Take care, now...oh, Doctor! Wait one second, I just thought of something, while I have you.

I think my hair is falling out.

Terminal Crankiness

It's been a tough week. If my staff ever decides to change careers, they should be well trained for work in a complaints department.

First there was Blanche, a fifty-something woman who's been my patient for years. Her rosacea flared up, so I wrote a prescription for an antibiotic to help her face for her daughter's upcoming wedding. Next day I got a request that I fax another script to one of those mail-order pharmacies somewhere in Outer Darkness where rent and wages are low. Two days later the mail-order place requested a clarification: which chemical salt of the medication did I want? (In thirty years no pharmacy has ever asked that before.) I faxed back my answer.

And now Blanche was berating my secretary loudly and at length because the mail-order place was still preparing her order. She demanded that we pay for overnight shipping to compensate for our sloppy incompetence. For good measure, she canceled her next appointment.

Asking us to pay for shipping was a new one. (A patient once did demand that I pay for dry-cleaning a dress when an ointment I'd prescribed got on it.) I called Blanche back, and left a polite voice mail message suggesting that she direct complaints of this nature to the mail-order pharmacy whose procedures were perhaps more pertinent than ours to her dilemma.

Later the same day Alfred came in, a slovenly and truculent man in his early seventies. His real concern was that we laser the age spots off his face. (You really can't tell a cosmetically-oriented patient by appearance.) Alfred had a slightly raised, red patch on his right cheek that seemed at an earlier visit to be a collection of blood vessels but had now developed a bit of texture. I explained that laser surgery would not work and suggested a light scraping procedure to both remove the spot and test it to rule out skin cancer.

Alfred would only agree to this if I guaranteed—in writing—that there would be no mark left afterward. I explained that I couldn't offer such a guarantee and why I felt it would be best to test the lesion, adding that leaving it there would guarantee he would still have a spot. "Oh, so now we're just speculating," he growled, and walked out.

And you have a nice day too, sir.

Next day was even better. My associate Megan, who has a soft manner and infinite patience, told me she had just endured a telephone tirade from a woman whose twenty-one-year-old daughter had fungal toenails. We had actually diagnosed this seven years earlier, offered the daughter the option of an oral antibiotic, and asked the mother to arrange for blood testing as a possible prelude to treatment.

They never got the testing done, and the daughter had been back several times over the years for other issues without ever raising the fungal concern. Megan heard out the mother patiently, spoke soothingly, and talked about treating with the antibiotic when the daughter returned from school in May.

"In my family we don't use generics," came the frosty reply.

I called the mother back. (She was in Florida with her daughter, on spring break.) I explained that generics can, indeed, be okay. "I had a bad experience with one," she retorted. I told her that we could certainly start antifungal treatment after this semester, if her daughter wanted us to. And so on. She sounded mollified.

The question, of course, is why now? After having fungal toenails for seven years, why did her daughter suddenly find it urgent to clear it up? What about all those visits in between, which spanned most of her adolescence?

People just get cranky, I suppose, and it was our misfortune to encounter three in a row. I guess I ought to make allowances for matrons aflutter in the run-up to their daughter's wedding, or for shlumpy gents who do indeed care deeply about their appearance, or for parents of excitable young ladies with acutely intolerable toenails, all of whom have decided to relieve their inner tension by beating up on me or my staff in full-throated arias of crankiness.

Only I'm feeling cranky myself just now, so I'm not in the mood for making allowances. You'll understand, won't you?

You won't? Too bad.

Life Gets in the Way

Patients don't call you back. Or, more precisely, patients call back when they want to, not when you want them to.

You know the drill. Harry is on the phone with another update on his hives. They're driving him crazy, and being a generous man he wants you to share the experience.

And so he calls once a day to tell you how his hives are. Today they are on his ears. Yesterday they were on his thighs. Last Friday they swelled his scalp up something awful.

Besides his observations, Harry wants you to comment on and support his speculations. He thinks maybe the hives are worse when he's hot, when he eats acid foods, when he watches the late news. What do you think?

And then one day Harry doesn't call, and you realize that he hasn't called in days. Could he be better? Or perhaps he got worse and consulted someone else? Was your hunch about additives on the mark, or was the dye a red herring? You call him with some trepidation (maybe he's mad) to ask what's up. He doesn't call back. Two years later Harry drops by with toenail fungus. The hives? Oh, he says, they went away. He doesn't remember exactly when.

It's hard to get better at what we do if we often can't find out how things develop. Why won't people get back to us?

Armchair analysts who ponder this question develop tidy lists of plausible reasons. The doctor was cold and overbearing. She used off-putting jargon, or seemed rushed. Health care is impersonal. It costs too much. Male doctors are patronizing and hegemonic. Whatever.

I have little doubt that explanations like these account for some fraction of poor follow-up, maybe ten percent. For the remainder I have a better explanation: life gets in the way.

I gained this insight at a practice marketing seminar. The presenter was a slick, short Californian with big hair. I learned from him that marketers have deep insight into their clients' minds. This is not because they are by nature especially intuitive people, just that sensitivity is their stock-in-trade. If they lack it, people don't buy what they're selling and they lose money.

After two intense days, Mr. Pompadour addressed the group with great earnestness:

"You agree that our ideas are good. You know they'll pay off for you. But if you don't implement them the minute you get back to your office, you never will. Life will get in the way."

Prosaic? Part of the spiel to close his own sale? Sure. But true nevertheless, and instructive too. Patients know it's in their best interests to contact you. They like you and appreciate your concern. They mean to call you back. They just don't get around to it.

So you tell your patient to inform you about medication side-effects. She doesn't call. At the next visit she says she stopped the cream after two days because it burned, and she never picked up the pills because she hates pills. She figured she'd tell you about it some other time.

You advise skin cancer patients to get annual checks to pick up new or recurrent lesions. They agree. You send them one reminder, then another. They don't show. Years later they come back. "Here for your annual?" you ask. "Not at all," they say. "There's this new spot that worries me…"

Irrational, even perverse? At times. But that's how people are. The worry that overcomes inertia and spurs their call is their worry, not yours. And by the way, are you yourself perhaps a little behind for that six-month checkup with your dentist?

When I speak to my medical students facing life in whichever aspect of the profession they choose, I advise them as follows:

If you don't much care whether a patient makes a return visit, fine. But if you really want them to come back, you had better be ready to do whatever it takes: cards, calls, e-mails, gumshoes. If you're not prepared to be bothersome and persistent, don't try to salve your professional conscience by telling yourself, "Well, they're adults, and I warned them." You know, or ought to know, better than that.

I Don't Have
Health Insurance

Stephen moved from Boston to New York to study opera, and supports himself by leading church choirs. He knows that because his father had melanoma, many moles put him at risk for that serious malignancy.

"I haven't been checked in several years," he admits. "But now that I'm back in school, I have health insurance."

Let's apply rational economic analysis to Stephen's behavior. He knows that melanoma is a dangerous cancer, that he is at risk for developing it, that regular checkups are his best hope for avoiding it. Beyond food, clothing, and shelter, he expends disposable income on various elective choices: travel, movies, restaurants, and so on.

But he won't pay to take action to save his life unless it's covered by health insurance.

Got that?

As every clinician knows, Stephen is not alone. Daily we meet people who won't take care of the acne that's making them miserable or the eczema that's driving them crazy until they have insurance, despite financial comfort or even affluence. They would never stint on quality or even elegance in clothes or food, but balk at a $25 co-pay for a brand-name drug, even if the generic is icky. There are the more extreme examples, like Myrna, who is on welfare but tells me she just had a nose job. "I know this doesn't make sense," she offers.

No and yes. The job of a clinician is to understand people, not complain about them. Hectoring patients ("You went to Bermuda, dintcha, so how come you won't spring for minocycline?") is both offensive and useless.

In 2002 Daniel Kahneman won the Nobel Prize in economics, for "having integrated insights from psychological research into economic behavior." According to a Princeton colleague, Kahneman's work showed that, "If people are not always capable of making rational decisions, then a lot of what economists had inferred on the basis of those assumptions really needed to be re-examined."

I know nothing about economics, but you really have to wonder about a field that gives someone a Nobel Prize for noticing that people don't always maximize their prospects by acting in accord with rational principles. No kidding.

I am not aiming for a Nobel (though I will graciously accept one if offered), but make bold to offer the following explanation for the irrational economic behavior under discussion. The universe of expenses is divided into three fiscal categories:

- Things I have to spend on or else I will die of starvation or overexposure.

- Things I don't absolutely need but I will spend on if I can afford it because no one else will do it for me.

- Things that somebody else will pay for; I am a chump if I pay for these myself even if I can swing it.

Back in pre-insurance days, people treated the doctor like the grocer, running up only the bills they felt they could handle. The very existence of health insurance does more than make health care affordable; it shifts medical expenses into another category altogether, one in which "I can" and "I can't" are replaced by "I don't need to" or even "I'm a fool if I do."

How else can one explain my online respondents, who would never dream of whining, "I can't afford a movie!" yet see nothing odd about describing their utter misery and adding, "I can't afford to see a doctor." (Really? For one visit?)

The erosion of health coverage in recent years has made physicians' lives somewhat easier in one respect. Nowadays people no longer assume that insurance covers everything, and are less offended to learn that a particular service or medication is considered cosmetic or otherwise not reimbursable.

In the ongoing debate over universal health insurance, it may be worth considering that health expenses are not like other outlays, the ones people will make if, according to balance sheet calculations, they can manage to afford. There's a difference that goes beyond bank balances between what patients can afford and what they want to afford, even if they know their lives are at stake.

Ask Stephen.

Bad News

We specialize in good news. You don't have a dread disease, we tell people. You aren't contagious or repulsive. That spot isn't cancer, and even if it is we can take care of it. Patients shower us with thanks and praise: *You make me feel so much better*, they say. *You are the best*.

But not this time.

I had seen Heather on Wednesday, a vibrant, self-confident young woman from out west with the milkiest, bone-white skin one could imagine. She spoke of plans for summer research and a career in science. She had a mole in her groin that was rubbing. I'd like to have it off before I go home, she said. Shave removal was quickly done. The test results would be of no interest, but I would let her know.

Her biopsy report reached my desk late Thursday afternoon. Melanoma, Clark Level IV, almost three millimeters thick.

Shock gave way to uncertainty. How to tell a young woman you hardly know troubling news for which she is totally unprepared, that she has a serious disease with a possibly grave prognosis.

Certainly not on the phone.

I called her cell. "Where are you?" I asked.

"I'm out walking a few blocks from your office," she said. I was relieved. "Come over right now, please," I said. "I have to talk to you."

Ten minutes later Heather sat in one of my exam rooms. A young man paced in the waiting area.

I faced her. "I don't have good news," I said. "The mole I took off yesterday turned out to be cancer."

Her eyes widened in terror. "What do you mean?" she said. "What kind of cancer?"

"Melanoma," I said. "This could be serious."

Heather started to weep. She said, "But that doesn't make any sense! Skin cancer is from the sun. I've never been in the sun. Never! This can't possibly be true," she said. "How can this be happening? Why is it happening to me? It isn't fair, it doesn't make sense!"

I agreed, of course, but this was not the time to say so, to say anything at all. Heather wept with agitation. I joined her, but just a little, out of decorum.

After a while, we spoke of steps to take. She had to call her parents. "My God," she said, "what am I going to tell them?" I offered to assist.

"It would be best to go home right away," I said, "not wait for classes to end." She would need the cancer removed, staged. "Further treatment might possibly be needed."

"Possibly!" she cried, her voice heavy with sarcasm, fear turning to fury.

I invited her friend in to console her. Dad did not answer. I gave Heather my cell number, so he could reach me later. Her friend joined us. The two embraced, alternating tears and laughter. They are very young.

Both soon left the office, our acquaintance intense but brief. I had barely met Heather, and wouldn't be seeing her again.

That evening and much of the next morning were taken up with logistics: explanations to parents, calls to doctors in Heather's hometown, e-mails of reports. She arranged to leave school, canceled summer research plans, rescheduled a flight home for prompt consultation with a surgical oncologist. Details are easier to confront than the enormity of what occasions them.

Why me? Why now? Every ill person asks these questions, but who can say? Why does my rash go away and come back? Why is it on my chin and not my forehead? Is it my food, my behavior, my genes? Is it my fault?

Never mind, we say, let's just try to make you better. Though we rarely know the whys of things, it usually doesn't matter that much.

But sometimes it does matter that much. Why should a young woman with her whole life before her be in mortal danger? As

Heather saw at once, it isn't fair, it isn't right, it makes no sense.

No, it doesn't. But there is little to do besides attend to logistics and leave to other counselors the job of helping her confront what no one can explain.

In any event, tomorrow another week begins. It will be pleasant to resume the routine of ordinary work, dispensing more of the good news in which we specialize.

A Purely Cosmetic Procedure

"Why on earth would you want to remove tattoos?"

When my colleagues learned that I remove tattoos in my practice, they were puzzled and skeptical. What motive could a physician have for doing that sort of thing, other than the obvious one—greed? Bad enough to use lasers (or other means) to rid patients of birthmarks, scars, or other defects of no functional significance.

We dismiss such concerns as "cosmetic," which is to say trivial and frivolous. In the medical world, a cosmetic problem is not "real," not something physicians should bother to diagnose, much less address. Insurers reinforce this definition in the most potent way possible: by reimbursing only for those problems physicians count as real. Foolish enough, then, to bother with marks that, however petty, are at least acts of nature. But tattoos? Do people who deform themselves deserve our ministrations to undo the predictable results of their own folly?

Some of my colleagues' questions sounded faint but clear class undertones. As one put it, lowering his voice a bit (although we were alone), "Do you really want the kind of patients who have tattoos?" That clientele is plainly not "our sort" of people. Who are these tattoo types, anyway? What motivates them? What are they after? Why do they mutilate themselves in the first place, and how will they react if treatment doesn't produce the results they expect? One never knows about these cosmetic sorts. They may be narcissistic, unrealistic. Their very concerns mark them as unhappy with themselves.

I was about fifteen, I guess. I grew up on the east side of town, the poorer side. Nobody paid much attention to what I was doing, so I was out on the streets by the time I was in ninth grade. You know—broken home, alcoholic father, Mom too busy trying to keep the house going to pay much attention to my sisters or me.

I don't remember exactly how it happened. Just one night a bunch of us got together and drove to a town downstate. One of my buddies said he knew a guy who had a tattoo parlor there, and we all had one put on. It didn't hurt too much. I remember the tattoo guy gave me a choice of designs. This skull tattoo he put here on my arm—I don't even think it's the one I picked, but it didn't matter, as long as I had one. You can see it when I wear a short-sleeved shirt.

My in-laws have been very nice. Really, they never mention it at all, but my father-in-law did say he would pay for it if I wanted it off. He's a big attorney downtown, and he's on the Board of Trustees at the university.

My wife grew up a lot different from the way I did. Like I said, I'm from the other side of the tracks and she's from the good part of town, where her folks still live. They have some house, you should see it. They give parties there all the time, for the attorneys in her dad's firm and for the Trustees at the university. And like I said, her family's awfully nice. They've always accepted me, ever since my wife brought me home to meet them.

And now I have a house of my own! It's small, two bedrooms. My wife and I use one, and the girls are in the other; one's three and the other's six months. I started my own business last year. It's going pretty well, but I still do some work for my old boss to help make the house payments. Between the two jobs, we'll be okay.

I look at myself and I can hardly believe it. Here I am, thirty-two years old, with a wife, two kids, a house, and my own business. I don't even recognize myself. When I was fifteen, I never pictured myself doing any of these things. I can't even really figure out how it all happened.

This tattoo on my arm, I guess it was a stupid thing to do, a kid thing. Whenever I look at it, it reminds me of who I was then. My wife and my in-laws look at it too, but like I said, they're too nice to say anything.

And then I look at who I am now. This tattoo reminds me where I came from. But I'm not the kind of person who would put a tattoo on, at least not anymore. And you know, sometimes I think maybe it isn't right for me to be taking it off like this. Maybe I don't deserve to forget where I come from.

During this soliloquy the laser beats out a rapid tattoo of its own. Each second a pulse of light, with a wavelength of 755 nanometers, carves several small disks out of the young man's unwanted skull tattoo. Seventeen years ago, in a group ritual with ancient roots and complex meanings, he had his class and social origins inscribed in his flesh. Now, crafting a new identity, he is having the brand expunged. The completed process will leave no scar, at least none anyone else can see.

His concerns, it goes without saying, are purely cosmetic. That is to say, they are airy and insubstantial, too trivial to engage the notice or warrant the attention of any self-respecting member of the healing profession.

Gifts

As a senior medical student I spent an outpatient December in the office of a suburban pediatrician who cared for the kids of many doctors. With the holidays approaching, he mused on the coming onslaught of gifts from people to whom he extended professional courtesy. Some would bring conventional stuff—candy, wine, and so forth. Others might aim for something more grandiose. Like the one who the year before had sent him a side of beef.

During the holiday season many people ponder the intricacies of giving and getting gifts. Knowing when and what to give, as well as how to accept, requires art and sensitivity. ("That's *exactly* what I wanted! How did you know?") Thankfully, such subtleties are less important for doctors, at least at work, now that health insurance and fixed co-payments have made most professional courtesy obsolete. I doubt many miss it. Professional relationships work best when objectivity isn't undercut by other considerations. Like presents.

Gifts haven't gone away, though. Some of my patients still like to bring presents. When Mrs. Serebrennikova hands me a box of chocolates covered in Cyrillic script and those funky Russian, ruby-red graphics, I protest that she really shouldn't have (though gently, so as not to offend). Bringing the gift clearly makes her happy, and my staff eats the chocolate.

Many of my Russians like to bring gifts. Besides chocolate, they present wine and other spirits. One Russian physician brought a bottle of Armenian vodka in a bottle whose odd shape I couldn't make any sense of until he showed me how to hold it: it was shaped like a boxing glove! I show it to houseguests, but it's just too weird for me to open. (Some time later I saw another vodka bottle from the former Soviet Union, this one shaped like a submachine gun.)

Other ethnic groups bring presents too. Mrs. Wong generally brings cookies from Chinatown, and sometimes tea. Pamela brings a loaf of Irish bread every time she comes for Botox. She says she knows how much I like it. I have no idea how she could know this, since I have never eaten an Irish bread, but I don't have the heart to tell her that. My head nurse Fiona O'Connor grew up in South Boston. (If you can't locate Southie on the physical and cultural map, check out Matt Damon in *Good Will Hunting*.) *Fiona* likes Irish bread, including Pamela's.

So far the examples I've given reflect varieties of ethnic expression and traditional patterns of gift-giving left over from old countries. Other presents can be personal expressions—authors bring in a copy of their latest book, musicians drop off a CD. One patient last week brought an art calendar her mother had illustrated. A very elderly gentleman came by a few years ago, and reminded me that I had seen him decades before, when I first went into practice. In his '90s, he was still busy making mobiles, and he brought me one. Because I couldn't bear to throw it out but had no idea what to do with it, I hung it behind a door for a long time. Eventually, like most such things, it went away.

Then some gifts, like their givers, are just, well, odd. One gent came a few years ago for a minor problem that cleared by the second visit. Before leaving he rather solemnly announced that he was so grateful for my intervention that he had purchased a gift. He then reached into a tin bucket he'd brought along and withdrew a short, green brush, the kind you use to wash dishes, and presented it to me. The price tag was still attached—forty-nine cents.

I was speechless. I still am. The gift brush sits on my windowsill, reminding me of the importance of going the extra mile for patients, of washing dishes, and of buying things on sale.

Happy Holidays!

Underwear

"My husband saw you two years ago," Karen said. "You made fun of him because his underwear was torn."

Well, I hope I didn't make fun of him. Most likely he stripped to his skivvies for a full-body check and found he hadn't heeded Mom's advice: Always wear nice underwear in case you're in an accident. Or at a dermatologist.

Clothes make the man, perhaps more so the woman. Suits and dresses tell the world what we want it to think of us and what we think of ourselves. Underwear speaks too, but what does it say? As physicians whose patients often disrobe, we are in a good position to ponder this vital question.

At bottom, underwear is silly. To my small grandson, saying "underpants" is the height of wit; just hearing the word brings gales of laughter. Grownups get more nuanced, of course, but underpants are still underpants.

Most men aren't self-conscious about undressing, but now and then a fellow looks sheepish as he drops his trousers and confesses that he isn't wearing any underwear, which by then is obvious.

Apparently omitting undies requires an apology.

Men's fashion is simpler than women's, but even guys have options these days. We used to have your two basic styles, briefs and boxers, but now there are a dozen or more. Boxers come adorned with many designs, some erotic, but most just decorative: bright plaids and polka dots nobody would wear on the outside (who picks these anyway? Women, I'd guess.); hobby symbols (golf clubs); flights of whimsy (Jack Daniels, Rocky and Bullwinkle).

And then, of course, there are designer logos. Everyone recalls the scene in *Back to the Future* when a new acquaintance from the 1950s calls Michael J. Fox "Calvin" because that's what it says on his butt. There actually was a time when conspicuous consumption didn't extend to the inconspicuous, but now a Google search serves up a dozen styles and forty different brands, from stylish to sexy, from Fruit of the Loom to aussieBum to the ubiquitous Joe Boxer, who seems to be everywhere, if you know where to look.

Wearing designer clothes or shoes sends a clear message about affluence and status, or at least our aspiration to these. But what does designer underwear say, and to whom? This question seems especially pertinent when people with designer stuff underneath often sport outer clothes that are nothing special.

For women, of course, underwear (along with many other things) is more complicated. To start with, women take fashion more seriously than men, which is why they're offered an even more dizzying array of underwear styles and brands to choose from. Then there is practicality: women's underwear may limit their choice of shorts, or it might show those awful panty lines. I'll never forget the young woman who called for help with her inflamed bum. She had just won a bikini contest. "To avoid panty lines we attach the bikinis with Krazy Glue," she explained, "which really burns when you pull them off." Ouch.

But most of all, for women far more than for men, underwear is associated with feelings of attractiveness and self-worth. This makes interpreting underwear choices all the more perplexing. Until I saw them for myself, for instance, I had no idea that Victoria's Secret makes thongs in extra large.

I've seen it said that women dress for themselves and each other, not for men. If so, exotic BVD's may have more meaning for underwearers than for observers, current or potential. In the same way, it's not uncommon for unkempt, out-of-shape types of both genders to swoop in out of left field and ask about Botox. You can't always guess what people bother about by their public image.

If anyone can divine what's going on in people's heads, though, it's the marketers. Who knows what secrets lurk in the hearts of Man, or Woman? Victoria knows but she's not telling, because her focus group results are proprietary. Her catalog, however, speaks volumes.

In the meantime, for us discretion is best. Marvel if you wish at underwear styles and designs. Ponder their meanings if you must. But just look at the rashes and moles and move on. In the end underpants are just underpants, and the deeper stuff is not our department.

The Pen

This is an old story. It happened on Memorial Day, 2008, when gas was four dollars a gallon and drug companies were still allowed to give you pens with their name on them.

My wife and I were in a Toyota dealership, planning to buy a Prius Hybrid. We hoped to save $300 a year on gas and make a powerful statement about our commitment to the planet.

The salesman told us that the Prius was such a hot car that they literally couldn't keep one on the lot. You had to wait weeks for delivery, and when it arrived they asked the customer to let it stay an extra day so prospective buyers could fondle the hood.

When he handed us pens to sign papers, I looked at mine with that momentary disorientation you get when you see something familiar in a strange context. Then it clicked.

"Excuse me," I asked the salesman, "but did you know your pen advertises a drug company that makes a vaccine against venereal warts?"

He didn't know, but he did turn several interesting colors.

How that pen got there will never be known. Maybe the dealership had diversified by putting a sexually transmitted disease clinic in the basement.

I Have Found the Answer

Last year a psychiatrist consulted me as a patient and brought some promotional material about Goji juice. He said this was a remarkable nutritional supplement and suggested I sell it in the office. As a distributor, he would get a percentage.

I read through the handsome brochures he left and listened to the accompanying CD. This presented a dozen testimonials by chiropractors, physicians, and naturopaths, all of whom ascribed an impressive array of health benefits to drinking the juice of the Goji berry. These included: anti-aging, better sleep, improved sexual function and mood, controlled blood pressure and blood sugar, more mobility and clarity of thought, and a stronger immune system with fewer colds. Other benefits included help with allergies, psoriasis, back problems, ADHD, Parkinson's disease, and restless leg syndrome.

In addition, the speakers reported cases of amazing regression of metastatic prostate and breast cancers, and disappearance of suicidal depression, sometimes in a matter of days.

It would be easy to be cynical about all this, and to see it as just another link in the grand tradition of mountebanks and quacks, where the greedy exploit the gullible. Cynicism is too easy, though, because it addresses only the question of why people want to sell Goji juice.

But why do people want to buy it? Even the best sales pitch won't work when people don't believe in what you're selling. Are they really prepared to accept that any one thing can cure so many unrelated conditions, not to mention cancel mortal diseases in no time? It appears that they are.

Analysis of the Goji sales approach shows several elements:

• Scientific credentials: All the speakers on the CD start by announcing their field of expertise: chiropractic, medical, hard-science, nutrition. Then they list their degrees: BA's in biology and nutrition, PhD's in biochemistry, MD's, diplomas in chiropractic or naturopathy. Their educational institutions range from regional schools you never heard of in the Midwest and Queensland, Australia to esteemed institutions like Sweden's Karolinska Institute and Harvard Medical School.

• Scientific trappings: Several start by saying how, as men and women of science, they were skeptical at first that Goji could be really all that good. Many claim they were impressed by the numerous articles ("more than fifty") in standard medical and scientific journals they found in online searches. (My own online search of the medical literature yields fifty-seven references from Japan, most by K Goji, others by J Goji, and a few by their less-prolific namesakes

A, H, N, and T.) Several Goji testimonials include long, scientific words, like "complex polysaccharides."

- <u>Ancient wisdom</u>: Supplementing this patina of science are invocations of ancient tradition; that Goji "has long been used in the Asian highlands," that it may explain the storied "longevity in the Far East," that it reflects "thousands of years of ancient traditions of Chinese and Ayurvedic medicine."

So this is how it is: If experts with relevant-sounding credentials use plausible words, many are prepared to at least consider that these authorities can give not just partial answers to small questions but comprehensive ones to large questions, indeed possibly to everything.

This dynamic is not limited to exotic Asian berries with silly names. Not long ago a friend showed me a best-seller by a physician on wrinkles, specifically how to prevent and get rid of them. I read it and wondered: Would anybody be prepared to accept that a single chemical, alpha-lipoic acid, can solve and reverse aging practically all by itself, even if several literature references say it's useful? Could anyone think that they can turn their life around in six weeks by eating salmon? Apparently they can. The doctor who says so is rich and famous.

Closer to home, would anyone think that a cleanser or moisturizer is superior and capable of heaven-knows-what just because a doctor's name is on the label? I guess so.

There were several comments among the Goji testimonials I found almost touching. One called Goji an "Elixir for the ages." Another said he was sure that Goji would have a "greater impact on world health" than anything else he could think of. And most poignant of all was the man who said,

"I have finally found the answer. The answer is Goji."

It's easy to mock this kind of thing, but the impulse underlying it is profound and pervasive. Life presents many problems, many complex and insoluble. That we all know this doesn't stop many of us from believing, or being prepared to believe, that someone, somewhere, has The Answer.

Who can have anything but sympathy for those of our patients who think that, as relevant experts, we must actually have it?

Remarks to the
Medical Youth Forum

Good evening. How many of you have heard the expression, "The doctor hung out his shingle"?
Nobody? Well, no surprise.

It's a pleasure to speak to a group like yours, high-schoolers from around the country interested in medicine. You are meeting speakers from all parts of the profession. My job as a practitioner here in town is to tell you my story. I hope you find hearing it useful, but your stories, however they develop, will be different from mine.

Hanging out a shingle once meant opening a medical practice. Picture a doctor setting up solo shop in his home and telling the world he's arrived by hanging a shingle with his name on it from a post on his lawn. You've never heard the expression because nobody goes into solo practice anymore, certainly not in his house.

Times change in unpredictable ways. In 1981 I took over the practice of a retiring dermatologist. As we met in his home-office, a converted garage, he sat across his desk and said, "You young people like to spend money on unnecessary things. Like secretaries." I smiled to myself and looked at him the way you are looking at me, which is how the next generation will someday look at you.

If you had told me thirty years ago that a doctor would need not just a telephone but a whole telecom system with voicemail, a network of computers, and an army of clerks to enter data, check insurance eligibility online, scan insurance cards and privacy disclaimers, and access electronic medical records, I would have thought you had landed from another planet. Voicemail? Computers? E-mail? Online? Not to mention PPO's, OSHA and HIPAA regulations, ICD-9 codes, or concierge practices—where you pay a doctor extra for the honor of having your phone calls returned. Nobody could have foreseen any of these novelties, and no one can predict developments thirty years from now. The only sure thing is that changes will happen, and in whatever profession you enter you will deal with them because you have to.

But there is one constant. Though technology advances and systems change, people don't.

Six years ago I spoke to students at this Forum and told them how I became a dermatologist. In college I majored in math, lost interest, didn't know what else to do, and followed a friend's advice that medicine might be a good choice. In medical school I chose pediatrics because the internists at my alma mater were intimidating and pediatricians were nice. Out of residency I took a job at a university-connected hospital, where my boss told me I needed "a gimmick" to stay in academics and proposed dermatology, which, in school, I had never encountered or thought of. I spent time with a dermatologist and pretended to be one myself until my hospital lost its university affiliation. Since there were no opportunities for pediatric practice in our town, my wife, three small children, and I moved up this way, where I retrained in dermatology.

Not a very well-considered decision, was it? The students I was addressing were miffed. They were expecting a more linear, perhaps inspirational, narrative, along the lines of: "I always wanted to cure skin disease and help humanity." But that's not how it was, and if you ask your parents and other adults how they got where they are, you will find that's not generally how it is.

But the punch line is that it turns out I do want to save humanity, at least one patient at a time; I do want to heal the sick and comfort the afflicted. But at your age, and for some time after, I didn't know it yet. At seventeen, what can you know about your life? You haven't lived it. But you will.

With opportunity, family support, hard work, and good luck, I was eventually able to figure out what I wanted to do, and to spend the rest of my professional life doing it. May you have similar fortune in whatever work you end up pursuing.

If you do join the medical profession, you will adapt to changes no one can anticipate. But however diseases evolve and therapies advance, people will continue to worry, to get sick, and to die. They will need your help to navigate their journey. That won't change, whether you tell the world you've arrived by launching a website or by hanging up a shingle on your front lawn.

Thank you for listening. I wish all of you success, contentment, and the very best of luck.

About the Author

Dr. Alan Rockoff was born in Uniontown, PA and grew up in the New York area, where he attended Yeshiva College and the Albert Einstein College of Medicine. After residency training in pediatrics, he studied dermatology in Boston and began practice in 1979. As Assistant Clinical Professor of Dermatology at the Tufts University School of Medicine, he has supervised senior medical students for thirty years. Dr. Rockoff writes a regular column for *Skin & Allergy News*, a monthly newspaper for practicing dermatologists. He and his wife Shuli live in Newtonville, MA. They have three children and seven grandchildren (so far).